Defying the PAINS
of GRAVITY

Defying the PAINS of GRAVITY

USING PROPER POSTURE TECHNIQUE

Jeff LaBianco, DPT, CSCS

iUniverse, Inc.
Bloomington

Defying the Pains of Gravity
Using Proper Posture Technique

iUniverse books may be ordered through booksellers or by contacting:

iUniverse
1663 Liberty Drive
Bloomington, IN 47403
www.iuniverse.com
1-800-Authors (1-800-288-4677)

ISBN: 978-1-4759-5713-6 (sc)
ISBN: 978-1-4759-5715-0 (hc)
ISBN: 978-1-4759-5714-3 (ebk)

Library of Congress Control Number: 2012919643

Printed in the United States of America

iUniverse rev. date: 10/26/2012

Contents

Section II

Preface

I wrote this book in order to provide the general public with a simple-to-understand guide on how to prevent and decrease joint pain through proper posture. I began writing this book about one year after practicing as a physical therapist. Many of my patients appreciate and understand the importance of proper posture as I explain it to them during their therapy sessions. They have asked me where they can find resources that illustrate these same concepts in an easy-to-understand manner. As I thought about it I could not give them any specific references. The books that I could cite were either too in-depth or too difficult to understand without formal education. So I decided that I would give them my own reference. After working with patients ranging from juveniles to geriatrics and diagnoses ranging from neck strains to strokes, I have detailed the essence of proper posture in this short, clear guide.

This book is divided into two sections. The first section provides the reader with an overview of how the body works as a whole, what causes postural deficits, and how one can effectively correct them. The second section provides specific workout protocols that combine key strength and stretching exercises to help maintain proper posture and flexibility. Though it may be tempting to jump to the exercise protocol section, I invite you to read this book from start to finish so that you can fully appreciate the body and its functioning.

Acknowledgments

I would like to give special thanks to all of my former patients. Without your dedication to improve and your thirst for knowledge about this subject matter, this book would not have been possible.

I would also like to thank my good friend Jasmine Vargas for modeling my book and my father Steve LaBianco for photographing my book. Thanks also go out to my former coworker and physical therapist Andrew Sullivan, my brother and pedorthist Scott LaBianco for critiquing my book, and to my current colleagues for their support.

Lastly, I would like to thank my family. Without your love and support I would not be in the position to write this book.

Introduction

The Three Causes of Discomfort

Have you ever noticed how many different positions we place ourselves in throughout the day? Whether you're sitting, standing, walking, or running, bending over to pick up an object or standing with arms outstretched while replacing a lightbulb, your body is turned, tied, and twisted in numerous positions. Luckily, each of us is built to withstand most of these daily stressors, but sometimes our bodies are pushed over the limit, leading to injury. There are three main causes of injury:

1. Repetitive movements
2. Traumatic movements
3. Prolonged insufficient positioning

Because we are subjected to daily tasks that drive us to perform movements over and over again, use improper body mechanics that cause pains and strains, and place ourselves in unnatural, damaging positions, we must be aware of these factors and act accordingly. By understanding how an injury is caused, and by simply thinking about the positions we place ourselves in, we have the means to prevent discomfort by changing our daily habits.

Chapter One

The Essence of Proper Posture

Posture. The dreaded P *word. Brings back memories doesn't it? "Put your shoulders back," your mother would insist as you slumped in your chair as a child. "Stand up straight," your teacher would whisper while you pledged allegiance to the flag. Well, believe it or not, they had a point. Posture is important! Maintaining proper posture helps prevent aches, pains, arthritis, degenerative changes, and even neurological dysfunctions.*

The reason why many individuals have so much difficulty keeping themselves in the correct position is related to a simple rule of physics. There is a force constantly pulling down on us—a force commonly known as gravity. So why wouldn't we slump down? It's easier than sitting up straight. We're designed to adapt to our surroundings, and because of this we take the path of least resistance, unconsciously allowing ourselves to slouch and fall into typical poor posture. The problem is that, when poor posture is sustained day in and day out, some of our tissue structures—including ligaments, tendons, and muscles—become weak and lengthened while others become weak and shortened. This unbalanced push-pull effect will eventually cause degenerative changes within our joints because our tissue structures will become unable to absorb the same amount of force they normally do when they are at their proper length.

The Key Players in Joint Protection

Cartilage, ligaments, tendons, and muscles naturally act as shock absorbers in our bodies. They help prevent damage to the bone structure of our joints as we locomote.

Our bodies contain two main types of cartilage. Hyaline cartilage surrounds every joint in our limbs. It is present at each end of our bones so that when bones connect to form a joint, they are able to glide over each other just as easily as a piece of ice sliding over a frozen pond. Thick, dense fibrocartilage is located between the vertebrae of the spine. This type of cartilage is responsible for preventing impact and allowing mobility throughout the spine.

Ligaments are short bands of tough, flexible, fibrous connective tissue that connect bone to bone. I like to refer to them as joint connectors. They aid in the stabilization and shock absorption of the joint. Tendons, which connect muscles to bones, are flexible but inelastic cords made up of strong fibrous collagen tissue. Each muscle contains one tendon on each end, and each tendon connects the muscle to small attachments on a bone. Most muscles in the body cross at least one joint, allowing us to move our trunk and limbs once the muscle is contracted.

These tissue structures are located around each joint and have a similar job as the shocks on a bike.

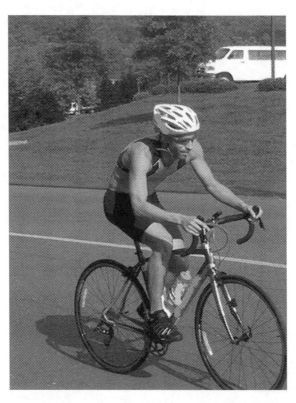

A good bike will have strong shocks that are able to absorb pounding forces as the rider bounces along the rough pavement. The shocks will attenuate the forces produced from the ground up, preventing damage to the bike frame and unwanted vibration. The tissues that surround your joints play the same shock-absorption role for your body.

Understanding Arthritis

Strong, well-positioned muscles will lead to optimal shock absorption. Muscles that are poorly positioned due to improper posture will be unable to absorb shock at their optimal capacity. This is detrimental to bone and joint health. Even though the cartilage is still able to perform its duty, putting the muscle at a mechanical disadvantage will place extra force onto the ligaments and onto the joints, leading to joint breakdown—in other words, arthritis.

Yes, the infamous arthritis! Have you ever wondered what arthritis really is? Well, before going any further, I need to clarify what type of arthritis I am talking about. The arthritis I discuss in this book is osteoarthritis, which is nothing more than joint degeneration. (This is not to be confused with rheumatoid arthritis, which is an autoimmune disease in which one's immune system mistakenly attacks healthy cells.)

That's right—arthritis is not some magical disease we must be confused about any longer. Arthritis is only found within joints. With the breakdown of hyaline cartilage, you don't have that smooth ice-on-ice texture within the joint that I described above. With arthritis, the bones that form the joint rub onto each other and cause degeneration. One thing to remember is that arthritis is a normal physiological process and we all get this wear and tear within our joints. Problems arise, however, when there is too much arthritis in the joint, resulting in discomfort and restricted motion. Having proper posture and knowing how to strengthen and stretch muscles through their full ranges of motion will help slow down the process of the inevitable arthritis.

The Cumulative Injury Cycle

I picked a box up from the floor and pulled my back. The box wasn't even heavy. Why does it hurt so much? This is a typical question I hear in the outpatient clinic. It's amazing how easily people hurt themselves. I have had patients (even some who work out at the gym at least three days a week) come in complaining of "stupid injuries" like pulling their backs after bending down to tie their shoes. So what's going on? Is it that people should be working out more than three times per week? Not necessarily. It is not that people are weak; the issue is that they have muscle imbalances. Their strength is in the wrong places, and they have set themselves up for muscle strain through prolonged insufficient positioning. The concept of pattern overload explains the problems with poorly positioned tissue structures in a little more detail.

Pattern overload arises when someone repeats the same pattern of motion over and over (whether actively or by remaining in a position for a prolonged period), which leads to overuse stress on the body. This concept will teach you how one's poor posture can cause internal physical problems.

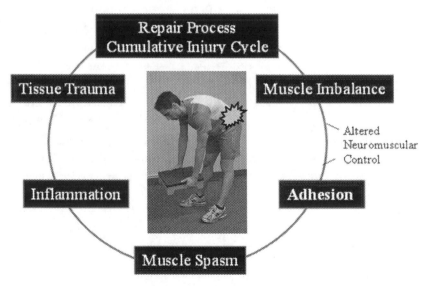

Let's take the example of picking an object up from the ground. A common action that gets people in trouble is using their backs instead of their lower bodies while bending forward. The length of your muscles will determine how efficiently you will perform the motion. If your back muscles become stretched and stressed, your body will recognize this stress within the connective tissue and will initiate a repair process known as the cumulative injury cycle. Tissue trauma or stressed tissue creates inflammation, which activates the body's pain receptors and initiates a protective mechanism. This protective mechanism increases muscle tension and causes muscle spasms to develop in order to protect the body from further harm. Highly active muscle spindles, sensory receptors within the belly of a muscle that detect changes in the length of the muscle, create microspasms that form adhesions or knots in the soft tissue.

These adhesions form a weak bond that decreases normal elasticity of the tissue; this then leads to muscle imbalance because less movement occurs in the muscle. When altered due to muscle imbalance, the joints will not move as fluidly, which can cause permanent structural changes, improper shock absorption, and increased potential for arthritis.

The Upper and Lower Extremity of the Body

Now that you understand how and why we *experience* pain, let's start exploring how the body functions as a whole so that we can learn how to *eliminate* pain.

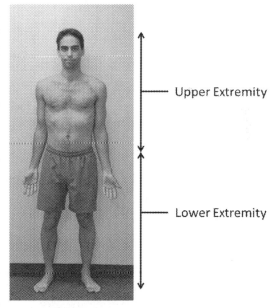

The term *posture* refers to a combination of body parts arranged in specific positions. Proper posture is the arrangement of those body parts in an optimal biomechanical position. In order to attain proper body mechanics, a person must place himself or herself in the appropriate position. Posture is like a collection of puzzle pieces, and the human skeletal structure is like a complicated puzzle. Different pieces, when put together correctly, show a complete and pleasant picture. If arranged improperly, the picture will become distorted, and the edges will not fit. Through knowledge, strength, and proper habits, we can reeducate our muscles to reposition our bodies from altered postures into proper postures similar to the way we would shift puzzle pieces around to fit correctly in their spaces.

In order to produce that appropriate and complete picture, we need to know what "pieces" or components make up posture. For ease of understanding, I divided the body into two major groups consisting of the upper extremity, anything above the waist, and the lower extremity, anything below the waist.

The Upper Extremity

We can sort the upper extremity into four body parts:

- Head
- Neck
- Shoulders
- Back

An important concept to understand is that all of our body components are connected to each other and affect each other through multi-joint muscle connections. When one joint changes position, it affects the position of the other components; so in order to keep optimal posture, we must assure that every component is in the ideal place.

The Lower Extremity

We can sort the lower extremity into five body parts:

- Hip
- Pelvis
- Knees
- Ankles
- Feet

Again, all of these components are directly or indirectly connected to each other, and they never work separately from one another.

The Spinal Column

Success depends on your backbone, not your wishbone. So, before we move on, let's briefly discuss a very important body component that extends through and connects the upper and the lower extremities: the spinal column. The spine is comprised of thirty-three small bones called vertebrae. These protect the spinal cord and support the body, allowing us to stand erect. Between each vertebra are discs made of fibrocartilage that act as shock absorbers, support the torso, and allow flexibility throughout the spine. Without these discs, there would be no motion in 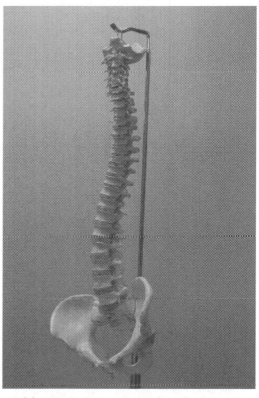 the spine, and the vertebrae would compress upon each other, causing extreme joint degeneration.

The spine is broken into five separate columns. The two lowermost columns, the sacral spine and coccyx bone, connect to the pelvis, which forms the hip. The other three consist of the cervical spinal column, the thoracic spinal column, and the lumbar spinal column. These are the main segments that allow both stability and mobility to occur throughout the spine.

The cervical spinal column is comprised of the seven vertebrae associated with the neck. These spinal vertebrae are smaller and more angled than the thoracic and lumbar vertebrae.

The small size and greater angle of these vertebrae allow for greater neck movement, compared to the back movement allowed by the thoracic and lumbar vertebrae.

The thoracic spinal column is comprised of the twelve vertebrae in the midback and torso. It connects the rest of the spine with the upper and lower extremity. This segment of the spine has the least movement out of the three main segments, but is just as important as the others. The ribs connect to the vertebrae in the back and to the sternum in the front of the body. The shoulder blades, which attach to the ribs, are part of the shoulder complex. These bony connections enforce the superior stability of the thoracic spine.

The lumbar spine is comprised of five vertebrae. These lumbar vertebrae are significantly larger than the cervical and thoracic vertebrae. Their position is also more neutral, allowing for greater rotation and movement to occur there than in the thoracic spine, but offering less freedom than in the cervical spine. The large vertebral bodies are constructed to accept and absorb the bulk of the ground forces and body weight. Since the cervical spine is only supporting the weight of your head, which weighs between about eight and twelve pounds, it will have more freedom of motion compared to the lumbar spine whose job is to support the majority of your body. Just feel for yourself! Rotate your head from side to side and compare that to rotating your trunk near your hips from side to side.

The Importance of the Thoracic Spine

I want to quickly touch upon the importance of the thoracic spine's motion. As described previously, the thoracic spine is connected to the upper and lower segments of the spine as well as the shoulder complex and can cause problems in these areas if not stretched properly. If the thoracic vertebrae are tight, movement in the thoracic column will be restricted, and because the body is very good at getting the motion it needs to perform a task, it will find extra motion in another joint. Since the cervical and lumbar spinal segments are closest to the thoracic spine, they will take up the motion that the thoracic spine cannot provide. If too much movement is placed on one particular joint, that joint can become hypermobile and overstressed.

With more mobility comes less stability, and less stability can lead to greater wear and tear of the joints. That's why it is important to keep the thoracic vertebrae properly stretched to allow for full and proportional spinal column function. Sitting thoracic mobilization is a common and simple do-it-yourself exercise for the thoracic spine that we will get to in the next chapter.

Common Symptoms Associated with Poor Posture

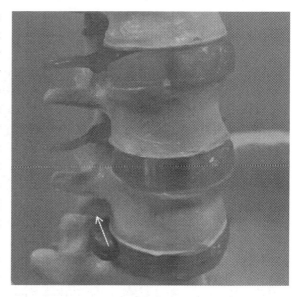

Many of my patients come into the clinic and tell me that their doctors told them they have sciatica. Okay. Now what? It seems many people know the word but do not understand the concept of this diagnosis. So let's review. Sciatica is a set of symptoms consisting of pain, numbness, and/or tingling caused by compression and/or irritation of one of five spinal nerve roots that form the sciatic nerve. Sciatica can occur from spinal stenosis, which is the narrowing of the spinal canal (the space through which the spinal cord runs). When this narrowing occurs it may cause cord compression and lead to the symptoms described above. But how does spinal stenosis occur? You guessed it—arthritis.

Sciatica can also occur from disc herniation. The disc can bulge back enough to push on and irritate a nerve, sending aggravating sensations past the lower back and into the buttocks and lower extremities, all the way down to the feet and toes. Before moving on, I'll review disc herniation because this is a common and annoying issue. Most poor postures, whether they occur while sitting or standing, place the spine in a more flexed or forward bent position. Even correct posture places a minimal but measurable stress on the vertebrae. These stresses on the vertebrae guide the movement of the disc. An improper constant forward position adds a compressive stress to the front of the disc and adds a stretching or tensile stress to the back of the disc.

The picture on the previous page illustrates the stresses that poor posture places on a disc. In this example we are looking at a disc herniation in the lumbar region. The arrow shows the disc material pushing against a lumbar nerve. This same concept can relate to a disc in the cervical or thoracic spine.

Think of the disc between each vertebra as being like a jelly doughnut and pretend that the vertebrae above and below the disc (the doughnut) are your hands. If you were to evenly squeeze down on the doughnut, the forces would compress the doughnut and disperse the jelly evenly.

Now, if you were to add the same amount of force, but squeeze down at only one end of that doughnut, the jelly would bulge out in the opposite direction. This would produce an uneven dispersion of force. With enough uneven force, the disc can herniate, adding pressure to the nerve endings of the spine resulting in pain, tingling, or numbness in the lower back.

Sciatica, though commonly associated with spinal stenosis and lumbar disc herniation, can also occur because the actual sciatic nerve is irritated or pinched due to a tight piriformis muscle or because the sciatic nerve is rubbing against the greater sciatic notch of the pelvic bone. This occurs in only about 10 percent of people with sciatica symptoms.

Similar sciatica-like pain running down the neck into the arms, hands, and fingers can be associated more commonly with cervical spinal stenosis, cervical spine disc herniation, and tight cervical musculature. Be aware that the pain, tingling, and numbness in the upper extremity is *not* sciatica; the sciatic nerve only exists in the lower extremity.

The Postural Control System

To finish up the chapter I would like to touch upon the fact that your posture is not just about your muscles. So what else is involved with posture? There are three main systems that are known as the postural control system. We just reviewed how ligaments, tendons, and muscle (which together form the skeletal muscle system) have a role in joint protection and postural control. But what actually controls our muscle movements? To discover this we need to look into the two other systems that make up the postural control system: the central nervous system and the sensory system. The central nervous system contains more nerves; they run throughout our bodies, sending and receiving signals to and from the brain via the spinal cord and controlling our muscle actions. Once a stimulus is sensed (sensation, vibration, pain, etc.), the nerves send a signal to the brain. A response from the brain is then relayed back to our skeletal muscles, instructing them to react to the stimulus by moving or holding the body in a certain position.

Trying to move our bodies without the central nervous system would be like trying to turn on a lightbulb without electricity. In addition to the many nerves, stretch reflexes are present which respond on a subconscious level to keep us in an upright posture.

The third system that controls posture is the sensory system. This system can be broken down into three components: the vision system, inner ear, and proprioceptors. These components allow us to keep our balance and stay in an upright position when moving or keeping still. Let's take a look at the eyes first. If you were to close your eyes and stand upright, you would need to concentrate more in order to keep your posture. Try it at home, and you may find yourself slightly swaying from side to side. Our inner ear deals with spatial orientation and sense of balance. Have you ever had an ear infection and felt dizzy because of it? That happened because the increase in fluid in your ear due to the infection adversely affected your inner ear. Proprioceptors located in our muscles allow us to have proprioception, the ability to sense the position, location, orientation, and movement of the body and its parts.

Chapter Two

Proper Sitting and the Ergonomically Correct Work Station

Static posture is any posture held for a prolonged amount of time. In order to stay in a static posture, one must maintain static postural control. This control is produced by the postural control system. Greater muscular control, which improves muscle strength and balance, in addition to proprioception and nerve connections, allows the body to remain in a proper static posture. This chapter explains how to sit properly throughout the day and lays out simple exercises that will improve the postural control system through simple stretches and active strengthening.

I am willing to bet that at least 60 percent of the people who will read this book, at one point or another, have had a job which required them to sit in a tight office space for most of the day. Conservatively speaking, a forty-hour workweek, not to mention overtime, takes up at least 50 percent of your daily life. Add to that the amount of time you spend at home sitting while watching TV, eating meals, reading the newspaper, and surfing the web. Don't forget commuting to and from work or, for business travelers, sitting in an airplane. That's a lot of sitting time! Sitting for an extended period of time in a position that adds physical stress to your body causes you to feel uncomfortable and reinforces poor posture. Sitting correctly is important. Doing so positions our muscles correctly, preventing discomfort and the risk of injury. Keeping that in mind, let's look at your sitting posture and take steps to improve it.

Guidelines for Proper Sitting Technique

Below are guidelines for proper sitting technique. Read through them and see if you can make any positive changes in your sitting posture.

1. Keep your gaze level (rather than looking up or down) in order to prevent unwanted stress on your neck.
2. Keep your chest up and out so that your collarbones are level. Doing this moves your shoulders back into their correct position.
3. Keep both feet flat on the floor. Do not cross your legs while in a seated position. Crossing your legs rotates your hips and puts unnecessary pressure on your lower back.
4. When seated in your chair, keep your feet flat on the floor with your knees bent at a 90-degree angle. This will take pressure off your knees and lower back.
5. Keep your rear end flat against your seat. Do not lean onto or favor one side more than the other. Leaning to one side will add stress to your lower back and can cause lower back pain.

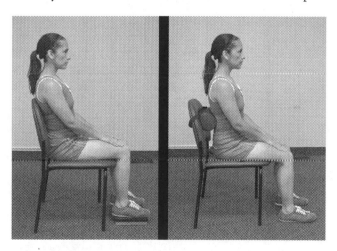

Four Common Postural Deficits

Now that you know how to sit correctly I would like to review four common postural errors and explain how to treat each of them. The person on the left shows proper posture; the person on the right demonstrates poor posture.

Proper Posture   Poor Posture

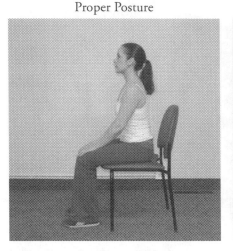 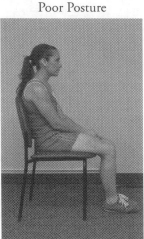

Forward Head Posture

The first main feature of poor posture is forward head posture. Keeping your head forwardly flexed throughout the day places additional stress upon the cervical spine, leading to neck pain. Picture your head as a bowling ball. Wouldn't it feel better to have it centered and supported over a strong spine than to have it extended out a few inches, pulling down on your neck? This is similar to the concept of holding an object close to your body rather than farther away. Picture yourself holding a gallon of milk. First, hold it close to your body and then hold it with an outstretched arm. Wouldn't the second position be harder to hold?

The situation is the same with your head. If your head is jutting forward, it will put much more strain on your neck than if you were to position it over your neck. Again, most of us are not intentionally forcing our heads forward; it is simply easier to let gravity pull us down rather than use our muscles to hold us up. Remember, though, since we subconsciously take the path of least resistance, we must *consciously* make an effort to avoid this, knowing that we will feel more comfortable and stronger in the long run.

Postural remedy:
Keep your head in a neutral position by aligning your ears with your shoulders while sticking your chest up and out.

What to stretch and strengthen:
- Stretch chest and strengthen neck

Exercise prescription plan: (Exercise descriptions located on the following pages)
- Doorway stretch or corner stretch
- Chin tucks

Forward Shoulder Posture

A second feature of poor posture is forward shoulder posture. This goes hand in hand with forward head posture because they are, like every joint in your body, connected. Forward shoulder posture is when the shoulders are pulled down by gravity, causing them to sink and fall forward. This position will overstretch and overstress the posterior (back of the) neck and the midback musculature while at the same time tightening up your chest musculature. Your posterior neck and midback extensors will remain weak due to extra muscle lengthening and your chest muscles will remain weak due to extra muscle shortening, further reinforcing this incorrect posture.

Postural remedy:
Pull your shoulders back by squeezing your shoulder blades together.

What to stretch and strengthen:
Stretch chest and strengthen back muscles

Exercise prescription plan: (Exercise descriptions located on the following pages)
- Doorway stretch or corner stretch
- Shoulder blade squeezes
- Chin tucks (cervical retractions)
- Backward shoulder shrugs.

Rounded Back Posture

Rounded back posture, also known as excessive thoracic kyphosis, is another common position you should avoid. *Thoracic kyphosis* is a term used to describe the normal convex curvature of the spine, but problems arise when this convex curve is magnified more than normal. Sitting with a rounded back will cause the spine to curve. With prolonged sitting in this posture, your back muscle will become lengthened and weak and will be unable to support your body in the upright posture. Your core stomach muscles will become shortened, further reinforcing this incorrect posture. If you are having trouble picturing this position, just think of elderly people that you have seen walking around slouched over; their bodies have physically adapted to the rounded back position. If you were to ask them to stand up straight, they would be physically unable to do so because their spines have been fused in that position for so long.

Postural Remedy:
Pull your trunk into a neutral position by bringing your chest and/or collar bones up and out.

What to stretch and strengthen:
Stretch the back and mobilize the thoracic spine

Exercise prescription plan: (Exercise descriptions located on the following pages)
- Thera Ball stretch
- Thoracic mobilizations (repeated extension in sitting)

Overextended Knees

Usually with this position, your knees are overextended because your feet are not supported on the ground. If your legs are hanging freely off a chair or are spread straight out, they begin to pull on your lower spine and upper body. That force further pulls on your spine, reinforcing the other three poor postural positions.

Postural remedy:
Support your feet with a step or a lift, which will place your knees at a 90-degree angle. This will relieve pressure on the lower spine and upper body.

What to stretch and strengthen:
Not applicable

Exercise prescription plan:
Not applicable

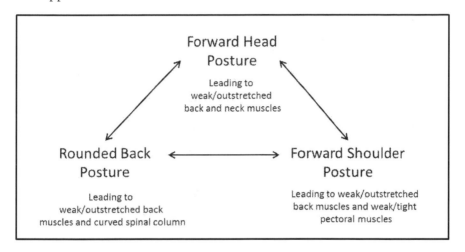

Note: Because the components of poor posture do not work separately from one another, we must remember that more than one deficit will most likely be present, and we must correct accordingly to form a collective overall proper posture.

Exercise Prescription Plan for Sitting Postural Deficits

Because our bodies have adapted to our postures throughout the years, very few individuals are able to reposition themselves in the correct posture and stay in that position. We need further reinforcement; and this is accomplished through strengthening loose musculature and stretching tight musculature. In the chart below, I have listed the specific exercise prescriptions that were noted in the previous section. The next few pages will describe how to successfully perform each exercise.

Dysfunction	*Correction*	*Exercises*
Forward shoulders	Stretch chest, strengthen back muscles	Doorway stretch, corner stretch, shoulder blade squeezes, chin tucks, backward shoulder shrugs
Rounded back posture (thoracic kyphosis)	Stretch back, mobilize thoracic spine	Thera Ball stretch, repeated extension in sitting,
Forward head posture	Strengthen neck and stretch chest	Chin tucks, doorway stretch
Overextended knees	Bend knees to 90 degrees while sitting	Postural correction: keep your knees bent at 90 degrees while sitting

Doorway Stretch

I enjoy this stretch because it targets the tight pectoral muscles that are present in many people who slouch in their chairs throughout the day. In addition to stretching the front chest musculature, this stretch places the shoulder blades in their proper anatomical position, reminding the body of where they should be. This stretch also improves the chest and midback proprioceptors. Find a doorway narrow enough to place both forearms against the sides of the wall. Place both forearms against the wall at shoulder height. Advance one leg through the doorway and bend that knee. Lean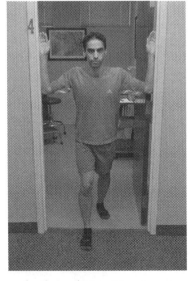

into the stretch and put some weight onto the bent knee. You want to feel mild discomfort *at most* during any stretch. Hold for thirty to sixty seconds three to four times.

Corner Stretch

Some of my patients have had difficulty with the doorway stretch because the doorways they have tried to use for the stretch are just too wide for their arms. If this is your situation, you can substitute the corner stretch. I do not find this stretch to be as effective as the doorway stretch, but it is the best alternative for those with short arm spans, and it will stretch your front musculature nonetheless. Stand in a corner with your forearms raised to shoulder height. Lean into your forearms until you feel a comfortable stretch across your chest. Hold for thirty to sixty seconds three to four times.

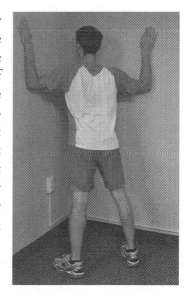

Shoulder Blade Squeezes

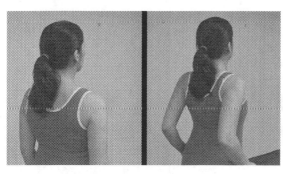

It's all in the name. Sit in a proper posture (see page 14) with your arms relaxed and by your side. Squeeze your shoulder blades together as if you were trying to crack a walnut between your shoulder blades. Perform this exercise at least twenty times making sure to hold for at least two seconds per squeeze.

Chin Tucks

Sit in a proper posture with your chest up and out. Next, retract or tuck your chin back. Do not bend your chin or neck while performing this movement. Any forward bending will only reinforce forward head posture. Performing 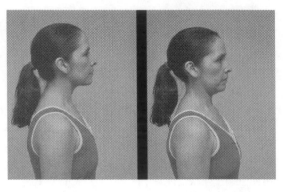 a chin tuck correctly involves a strictly horizontal motion. Imagine that a metal rod is attached to the top of your head. This rod prevents you from bending up or down. Now, just glide your head backward. Perform this movement for three sets of ten or until your neck begins to feel loose.

Backward Shoulder Shrugs

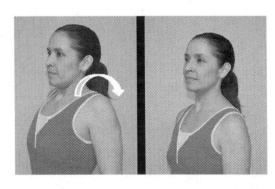 This exercise will help loosen up your shoulders and upper spine. Begin by raising both shoulders up at the same time; then slowly round them backward. Perform three sets of ten or continue until your shoulders begin to loosen up.

Supine Midback Stretch

This exercise is ideal for stretching out the midback, which, when tight, prevents you from keeping your chest up and out while sitting. Start by lying supine (on your back) on a rounded object that will stretch out your back such as a Thera Ball (Swiss ball). Hold this position for two to five minutes. In time you will be able to hold this position for longer amounts of time, allowing for greater flexibility in the whole spine.

You can also lie back on a foam roll, purchase a device called Back Magic, or even simply bunch up some pillows.

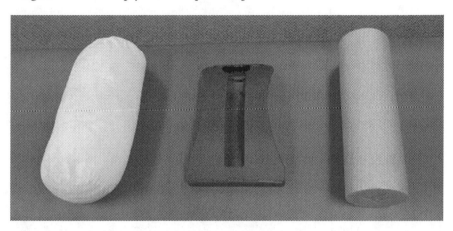

Thoracic Mobilizations (Repeated Extension in Sitting)

Start by sitting on a chair. Interlock your hands behind your head and gently bend backward into the back of the chair. Perform three sets of ten or continue until your midback feels loose.

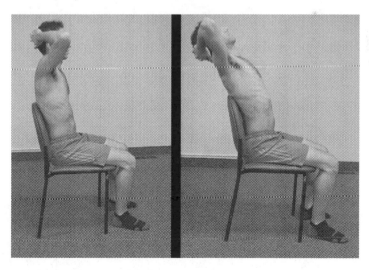

Postural Maintenance

How many of you get up and move around throughout the day? If you don't, it's time to get your rear into gear. Since sitting places the spine in a flexion bias, it's important to get out of that flexed position once in a while. It is optimal to do this every hour. This can be done by walking around the office for a few minutes and performing simple back extension exercises. Listed below are three simple back extension exercises. The first one is ideal for the workplace environment and the second two are more suitable for home. Though I'm sure some of you daredevils out there can brave the latter two exercises while at the office if need be.

1. Back extension while standing
2. Stomach lying on elbows
3. Stomach lying press-ups

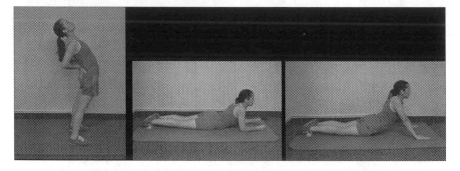

The neck and midthoracic spine should not be ignored. Shoulder blade squeezes, chin tucks, and the doorway stretch described in the previous section are ideal exercises.

Getting up and out of your seat every hour or so will allow you to stretch out your joints and will give you the opportunity to reassess and readjust your posture every time you sit back down.

I would like to share a simple self-correct technique with you. The great part is it only takes a few seconds to perform. First, get into a poor posture! That's right, *a poor posture*! Once you are in this position, sit up as straight as possible by bringing your chest up and out. Become aware of your upright and rigid posture. Once you have sustained this position for a few seconds, slightly relax your posture by lowering your chest and relaxing your back muscles by about 10 percent. You should feel as though you are sitting upright, but not so much that you are straining to keep yourself there.

We Are Three Dimensional

We've stretched out the lower, mid, and upper back, including the neck, but are we forgetting anything else? I would think so. We are three dimensional and can perform thousands of different movements throughout the day. As we function through our daily lives, our bodies moves through three planes of motion. We move forward and back in the sagittal plane. We move side to side in the frontal plane, and we are able to rotate in the transverse plane. Because we move in all three planes it is important to stay flexible in all three planes of motion.

I do understand that many people are very busy at work and time is limited. That's why I'm going to leave you with three important exercises that will assure improved and sustained motion in the side to side and rotational planes.

Trunk Rotation (Hip Circles)

These exercises will loosen up the hip and lower back muscles without putting excessive strain on any of the back musculature. Begin by standing with your hands on your hips and your feet spread slightly wider than your shoulders. Slowly and gently make a circle with your hips in a clockwise direction ten times. Then repeat this in a counterclockwise direction ten times.

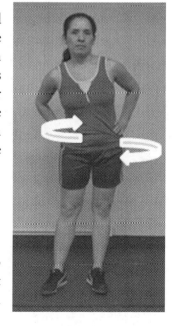

Trunk Rotation (Trunk Twists)

This type of trunk rotation is similar to the hip circle trunk rotation described above, except this time you will be moving your trunk on

23

your hips by slowly rotating your trunk from side to side. Perform this exercise ten times on each side.

Lateral Bending (Hip Side Bend)

This exercise will also loosen up the hip and lower back muscles without putting excessive strain on any of the back musculature. Begin by standing with your arms out to the side and your feet spread slightly wider than your shoulders. Bend to the left, sliding your hand down your lower extremity while at the same time shifting your weight onto the left foot. Then bend to the right, sliding your hand down your lower extremity while shifting your weight to the right foot. Perform ten times on each side.

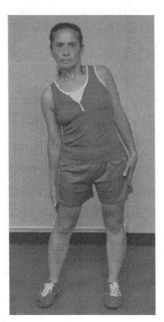

The Ergonomically Correct Workstation

On a clutter scale from zero to ten, (zero being no clutter and ten being as though a bomb went off in your office), what rating would you give your workstation? Some of us have messy desks, and as irrelevant or silly as it might sound, that clutter may affect you in a negative way. A well-ordered workstation will lead to continued postural improvement. Let's break down the different elements of a proper workstation.

Position Your Computer Correctly

First, you'll want to be able to look straight ahead and see your computer screen while your neck is upright in the field of vision; your line of sight should be horizontal to the middle of the monitor. If your computer is too low you can place reams of paper under the monitor in order to raise it to your eye level.

Position Your Body Correctly

You do not want to move your neck forward, bend your neck down, or lean from side to side in your chair. If you are in a position that causes you to twist or turn while looking at your computer, this will place increased stress on your joints, which may lead to pain, joint stiffness, and muscular weakness.

Maintain Proper Wrist Control

While typing, make sure your wrists are in a neutral position while resting on the keyboard. Flexing or extending your wrists increases the compressive forces on the joints, which may then lead to impairments such as pain, numbness, and tingling—and can result in more serious issues such as tendonitis or carpal tunnel syndrome.

Position Your Telephone Wisely

Your telephone is also an important tool in the workplace and should be placed in the most strategic position possible. Place the phone on the side of your nondominant hand so that you will have easy access to write messages with your dominant hand. Better yet, if you are frequently on the phone, I recommend wearing a headset. This will decrease the temptation to hold the phone against your shoulder, which can cause unnecessary cervical strain.

Sit Correctly

See the guidelines to proper sitting posture on page 13.

Remember Proper Back Support

Proper back support should also be attained with the addition of a lumbar roll to increase lumbar extension and prevent posterior compressive disk forces. If you do not have a lumbar roll, you can roll up a towel to about two inches in thickness and place it behind the small of your back.

The Dreaded Commute

Finally, your workday is over, and it's time to go home! So what do you do? You get into your car and sit for another twenty to thirty minutes. Statistics show that the average daily drive time nationwide is 24.3 minutes; and for many people, commuting time is much more than this. Sitting incorrectly for almost a half an hour can have a negative effect on your body.

Helpful hints for travelling in a car:

- Remove any objects in your back pockets. This will take pressure off your hips and lower back.
- Leave space between the back of your knees and the edge of your seat.
- Get as close to the steering wheel as comfortably possible. This will allow you to sit up straight and keep your knees in line with your hips.
- Use built-in lumbar support, or if your car doesn't have that, place a towel roll behind the small of your back or purchase a lumbar roll/support.

How many of you fly frequently? Those of you who do can certainly understand why airplane seats are notorious for causing neck and lower back pain. They are nonsupportive and uncomfortable, which increases the chances of sitting in a poor posture.

Helpful hints for travelling in an airplane:

- Bring neck and back support. Lumbar supports and neck supports are easy to find at local stores.
- If you do not have neck or back support of your own, put airplane pillows behind your back and neck.
- Get out of your seat and move around about every hour or so in order to keep your muscles limber.
- Perform in-flight exercises: arm raises, chin tucks, backward shoulder shrugs, and shoulder blade squeezes.

Chapter Three

Proper Standing Technique and Lying Postures

Standing postures place the lower spine in an extension-biased position. I believe this is less of a problem than having the spine in a flexed sitting position all day because most daily activities place you in a flexed posture.

Let's take a quick look at a normal day. You start bending forward from waking up in the morning until going to sleep at night while brushing your teeth, sitting on the toilet, bending over to put on clothing and shoes, leaning forward while washing dishes, cooking, sitting for meals, sitting on your sofa while watching TV and relaxing. Standing is helpful in offsetting this forward flexion movement. Only those who have occupations that maximally extend the spine day in and day out have symptoms due to overextension; this might include painters, electricians, construction workers, and gutter cleaners who perform work overhead.

Because many people have poor posture in standing, the normal extension is diminished, and the slouched forward position is increased due to poor standing. Our friend gravity can pull our bodies down, leading to flexed posture once again and to the symptoms described in the previous chapters. So it is important to learn the proper way to stand, just like proper sitting posture, in order to prevent unwanted pain.

Guidelines for Proper Standing Technique

Below are guidelines for proper standing technique. Read through them and see if you can make any positive changes in your standing posture.

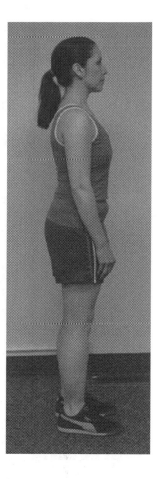

1. Keep your eyes facing forward. Do not tilt your head up or down. This will help prevent unwanted stress on your neck.
2. Your ears should be in line with your shoulders. Do not push shoulders forward in order to compensate, but instead pull your head back.
3. Keep your chest up and out so that your collar bones are facing horizontal (just as in sitting). By doing this your shoulders will move back into the correct position.
5. Your shoulders should be square with the rest of the body and your arms should rest comfortably by your sides.
6. Your hips should be even centered so if someone were to put a level across the right hip to the left hip it would be completely even.
7. Your knees should be straight and unbent, with both kneecaps facing forward.
8. Your feet should be flat on the ground and shoulder-width apart to provide a comfortable base of support.

Three Common Poor Postures

There are three common poor postures present in the standing position; they are caused by muscles being either too tight or too loose. Let's take a look.

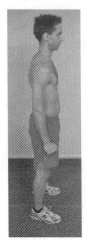 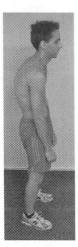 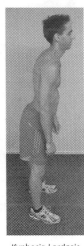 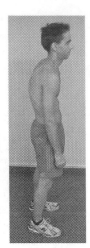

Normal Posture   Swayback Posture   Kyphosis-Lordosis   Flatback Posture
                                      Posture

Normal Posture

All muscles are working together without any muscle imbalances.
    See "guidelines for proper standing technique"

Swayback Posture

Swayback posture is characterized by a forward displacement of the hips. If you were to draw a vertical line upward from the front of the anklebones of someone standing in this posture, his or her hips would be in front of this line. The upper back is displaced backward in this posture in order to counter balance the forward position of the hips. People with this type of posture will have weak gluteal (backside) muscles. This type of posture is common in both men and women.

Postural remedy
Pull hips back by tightening up your stomach muscles and by pulling the small of your back backward.

What to stretch and strengthen:
Stretch the chest, stretch front hip, mobilize the thoracic spine, and strengthen mid back and gluteal muscles

Exercise prescription plan:
- Doorway or corner stretch
- Thoracic mobilizations (repeated extension in sitting)
- Shoulder blade squeezes
- Bridges
- Side-lying sweeps

Bridges

This exercise is ideal for strengthening the gluteal (backside) muscles and for stretching the front hip muscles. To perform this exercise, lie on your back with both knees bent at 45 degrees having your feet resting on the floor. Lift your backside about four to six inches off the ground. Hold this position for about two seconds and then slowly bring your backside back onto the ground. Perform this exercise for three sets of ten.

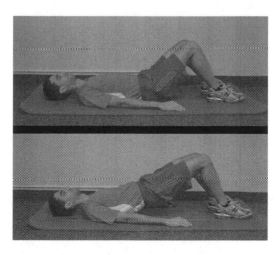

Side-Lying Sweeps

This exercise targets the external rotators, abductors, and extensors of your hips and is a very beneficial exercise to help strengthen them. Start by lying on your side.

Keep your body straight from your head to your toes. This exercise consists of three movements, which are performed simultaneously. The first movement is raising your leg up toward the ceiling, making sure that your knee is locked. For the second movement rotate your hip outward so that your toes point toward the ceiling. The third movement is slightly extending your hip or bringing your leg back. Perform these three movements at the same time. Then bring your leg back to the side-lying position. Perform three sets of ten on each leg.

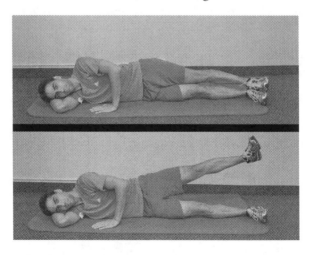

Kyphosis-Lordosis Posture

The kyphosis-lordosis posture consists of a forward head posture, thoracic kyphosis, and lower-back deep lordosis. The pelvis is also tipped forward in an anterior pelvic tilt.

Postural remedy
Pull hips back by tightening up your stomach muscles and pulling the small of your back backward. Also correct thoracic kyphosis posture as detailed in the upcoming chart.

What to stretch and strengthen:
Stretch chest, front hips, mobilize thoracic spine and strengthen neck

Exercise prescription plan:
- Corner stretch or doorway stretch
- Standing front hip stretch
- Thoracic mobilizations (repeated extension in sitting)
- Chin tucks

Flat Back Posture

This type of posture is characterized by a flat lower back, forward head posture, an increased curve in the neck, forward shoulder posture; also, the chest falls forward, and the back straightens out and stays flat, down to the lumbar spine. The pelvis is tilted under in a posterior pelvic tilt, and the knees are locked. This type of posture is common in both men and women.

Postural remedy
Correct forward head posture, forward shoulder posture, and hyperextended knees by following the instructions in the chart below.

What to stretch and strengthen:
Stretch chest and strengthen neck and back muscles

Exercise prescription plan:
- Doorway stretch or corner stretch
- Shoulder blade squeezes
- Backward shoulder shrugs
- Chin tucks

Commonalities between Standing Postures

As you look at the previous pictures, you can see that certain deficits are common to each poor posture. Forward head posture, rounded back posture, and hyperextended knees are present in each postural dysfunction.

These sound familiar, don't they? These are the same common postural deficits found in sitting. Remember that, because our bodies have adapted to these poor postures throughout the years, very few individuals are able to reposition themselves in the correct posture and stay that way. We need further reinforcement, which is accomplished through strengthening loose musculature and stretching tight musculature. The chart below lists specific exercises that will help with this.

Correcting Standing Postural Dysfunctions through Stretching and Strengthening

Dysfunction	Correction	Exercises
Forward head posture	Strengthen neck and stretch chest	Chin tucks, doorway stretch
Rounded back posture (thoracic kyphosis)	Stretch back, stretch thoracic spine	Thera Ball stretch, shoulder blade squeeze, repeated extension in sitting,
Hyperextended knees	Lengthen hamstring muscles	Hamstring stretch

Forward Head Posture

Perform doorway stretch and chin tuck exercises.

Rounded Back Posture

Perform shoulder blade squeeze, Thera Ball stretch, and repeated extension in sitting exercises.

Hyperextended Knees

Perform the hamstring stretches described on next page.

Hamstring stretches

There are many ways to stretch the hamstrings. The hamstrings are located in the back of the upper leg and are important muscles to keep limber because they have attachments to the hip, which are directly related to motion and flexibility of the spine. They also reinforce proper walking and bending technique. You want to have about 90 degrees of pure passive hamstring motion. Too much can provide excessive movement, which may lead to hip and lower back issues if your muscles are not strong enough in those end ranges. I will review a few stretches that I have found to be most beneficial.

Standing hamstring stretch

This is an easy-to-do stretch that can be performed just about anywhere. In addition to the hamstring muscle, this stretch stretches the gluteal muscles as well as the small lower back and midback muscles, known as the erector spinae group.

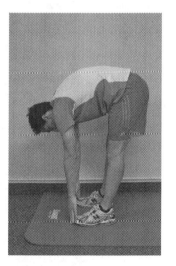

Start in a standing position, with your feet about six inches apart from each other. Slowly bend down with your arms outstretched and touch your toes keeping your legs straight. If you are unable to touch your toes, go as far down as you can until you feel a mild stretch in your hamstrings. Do not bounce. Bouncing up and down increases the risk for injury. If you want to target the inner hamstring muscles, perform the same exercises, but now spread your feet apart, about two to three feet, while pointing your toes out.

Hamstring towel stretch

This stretch allows all of your lower extremity muscles to relax. You passively stretch your hamstrings without needing to fire your front quad and hip flexor muscles as you need to do in order to bend in the first hamstring stretch. This stretch is probably more feasible to do at home unless you are feeling ambitious at work.

Lie down on your back and bend your nonstretching leg to about 45 degrees. This will prevent any chance of back pain during the exercise. Wrap a towel around the foot of the leg you will be stretching. With your leg straight, pull up on the towel and slowly raise your leg as high as you can just to the point where you feel a comfortable stretch with mild to moderate discomfort. Hold for thirty seconds and perform four times. (Note: You can substitute the towel with a dog leash, belt, jump rope, etc.)

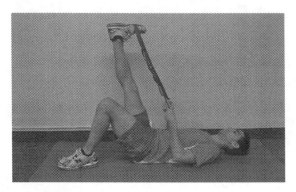

Sitting hamstring stretch

This is a nice stretch to perform because in addition to stretching your hamstrings you are targeting necessary lower back musculature such as the erector spinae group and the quadratus lumborum.

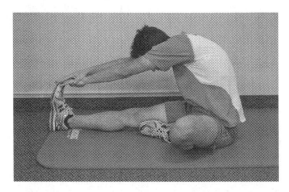

Start by sitting on the floor with your legs straight out in front of you. Keep the stretching leg straight and bend the nonstretching leg toward your groin so that the bottom of your foot is against the inner thigh of the stretching leg. Once in this position, gently lean forward with one hand outstretched over the other and reach for your toes. Stretch to the point where you feel a mild to moderate stretch. Perform this stretch four times, holding for thirty seconds each time.

Note: If this stretch aggravates your back, you can substitute bending forward and using a towel to pull your foot toward you. This substitution will not target your lower back muscles.

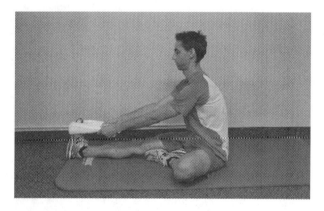

Standing Self-Correct Technique

Just like with sitting, reassessing your posture while standing for long periods of time is important. First, stand up as straight as possible by bringing your collarbones up and out. After sustaining this position for a few seconds, slightly relax your posture by lowering your chest and relaxing your back muscles by about 10 percent. This new position will place you in the proper standing posture. You should feel as though you are standing upright without straining to stay there. In time you will be able to sustain this position with less effort.

Three Common Sleeping Postures

A good laugh and a long sleep are the best cures in the doctor's book. Sleeping is one of the most beneficial things we can do in our lives to stay healthy. Sleeping allows our bodies to heal and recover from our stressors and daily activities. We spend about one third of our lives sleeping! There are three common sleeping positions we place ourselves in throughout the night. Each one places the spine in a slightly different position, and each position places stress on different parts of the spine. Like sitting or standing, lying down can add a flexion bias or an extension bias to the spine. Many people have different theories about the optimum sleeping position, and the position you sleep in can directly affect how you feel the following day. If you are someone who wakes up in the morning with neck or back pain, it would be beneficial to determine what sleeping position causes this pain. Uncovering what position causes you pain will enable you to correct it in the future. Let's look at three common sleeping positions and the mechanics involved.

1) Back lying
2) Stomach lying
3) Side lying

Back Lying (Supine)

Lying on your back places the spine in a slightly flexed position. This is because gravity pulls the front of the vertebrae to the back in an anterior-posterior direction.

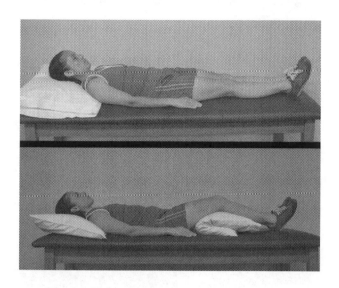

Some people with respiratory issues have difficulty lying in this position. People with respiratory issues may choose to prop themselves up with pillows. But remember, once pillows are added, the position changes, and changing the position changes the forces placed upon the spine. Propping pillows up against one's back will increase a flexed spine posture. This position is similar to the seated position; this is not necessarily bad. You just want to make sure you are not propping up too many pillows and falling into an excessive flexed posture for hours at a time. Excessive flexed posture will bring your neck forward and curve your spine.

If you find yourself propped up against pillows and complaining of neck or back pain, reassess your sleeping posture. It may be that you have too many pillows behind your head. Of course it is very hard to get out of a comfortable sleeping position. So in order to treat your pain and get into a better sleeping position, change the position slowly. Decrease the number of pillows one at a time each night. If your pain lessens but is still present, take another pillow out every few days until you are comfortable and able to sleep through the night.

Stomach Lying (Prone)

Lying prone (on your stomach) places the spine in a slightly extended position. This is because gravity pulls the back of the vertebrae to the front in a posterior-anterior direction.

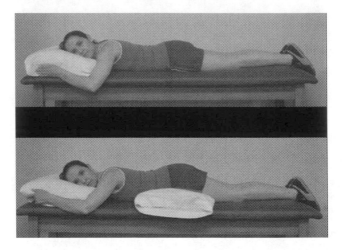

This position would be best to sleep in if you suffer from low back pain due to excessive sitting, bending forward, driving, or working at jobs in which you are in a flexed position. Sleeping in a slightly extended position will help offset your daily flexed postural positions. Although helpful in that sense, some people do not tolerate this position well.

Stomach lying causes a person to rotate his or her neck to one side which may add extra strain to the tissue of the cervical vertebrae because the neck is rotated to or near its maximum range of motion. Some people also experience headaches and dizziness due to the excessive cervical rotation and complaints of parasthesia (tingling) in their arms after a prolonged period of time. In addition to that, stomach lying may cause digestive issues.

Side Lying

Lying on one's side is a popular sleeping position. Side lying slightly curves the spine toward the side you are lying on.

If you have pain on the left side of your back, you may want to lie on your left side in order to close down the spine and push disc content or tight tissue structures back into the correct position. Also, if you experience back pain while lying on your side, instead of switching positions (which is very hard to accomplish if you've been sleeping that way for years), try folding a pillow and putting it between your knees. This will take stress off the curved spine.

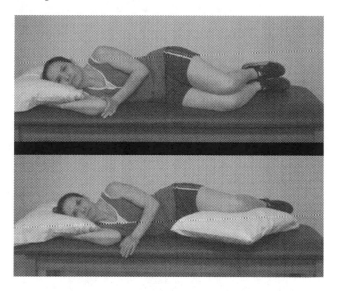

The Importance of Sleep

The Harvard Women's Health Watch suggests six reasons to get enough sleep:

Learning and Memory

Sleep helps the brain commit new information to memory through a process called memory consolidation. Studies show that people who'd slept after learning how to complete a task did better on that task later.

Metabolism and Weight

Chronic sleep deprivation may lead to weight gain by affecting the way our bodies process and store carbohydrates, and by altering levels of the hormones that affect appetite.

Safety

Lack of sleep increases the odds of falling asleep during the daytime. This may cause accidents and mistakes on the job such as medical errors or air traffic mishaps.

Mood

Decreased sleep may result in irritability, impatience, and the inability to concentrate. Too little sleep can also leave you too tired to do the things you like to do.

Cardiovascular Health

Serious sleep deficit has been linked to hypertension, increased stress hormone levels, and irregular heartbeat.

Disease

Sleep deprivation alters immune function. Adequate sleep may also help fight cancer.

Mattress Surface

Have you ever had an uncomfortable mattress? This can make a big difference when it comes to sleeping. Choosing a proper mattress is an important part of ensuring comfortable sleep. I would like to review a few keys points regarding the effects that hard and soft mattresses have on the body. A hard mattress surface has little cushioning, which can be uncomfortable for people with arthritis, rheumatoid arthritis, insomnia, bursitis (inflammation of the fluid-filled sacs that lie between tendon and skin and tendon and bone), and spondylitis (degeneration of the joints between the spinal vertebrae).

A hard mattress adds lateral stress to the lumbar spine for side sleepers and compresses the shoulder. They also flatten the thoracic spine in back sleepers, causing irritation in the midback. Mattresses that are too soft sacrifice postural alignment and add pressure and stress to the spine.

A mattress should be firm enough to prevent you from sinking but soft enough to conform to the normal curves of your body. Your spine should be in a natural balanced position. A mattress that is supportive and comfortable will allow your back to rest and rejuvenate during the night.

Mattresses vary widely in firmness, and with new and improved technology, there are many mattress choices. I recommend going to a mattress professional and choosing the firmness that best fits your needs. The only true test is the self-test. Lie on different mattresses and see what feels most comfortable.

Chapter Four

Dynamic Movements: Walking, Bending, and Lifting

Dynamic posture refers to postures in which the body or the extremities of the body are moving. These include walking, lifting, and bending. In order to have proper dynamic posture, you need to have an adequate range of motion while performing the specific task. You will also need adequate muscle strength to allow muscles to respond to various speeds and forces as they are stressed at different lengths throughout a task. This chapter will discuss the proper movement patterns and techniques for walking, bending, and lifting.

How far do you walk in a day? Do you ever think about it? Well, in this chapter I'm not only going to have you think about how far you walk, but also how *well* you walk. Walking, also known as ambulation, is a complex movement that requires the operation of many different muscle groups. The term *gait* refers to the manner or form in which one walks. A whole book can be written about walking and gait, but I will review just the main points here.

Guidelines to Proper Walking Technique

Walking is natural, and we don't need to think about how we walk; however, if we step back and think about how to walk, it will help improve posture and decrease chances of injury. Let's take a quick look at two key components of walking that will help assess and correct your walking posture.

Stand Up Straight

- Stand tall and straight with your chest up and out.
- Keep your eyes looking forward.
- Position your head so that your chin is parallel to the ground and your ears are in line with your shoulders.
- Keep your shoulders relaxed.
- Let your arms hang freely, keeping your hands relaxed and open.
- Keep your abdominal muscles firm by sucking in your stomach.

Begin Walking

- Allow your heel to strike the ground first and roll your step from heel to toe.
- Push off with your toe.
- Bring your opposite back leg forward to perform another heel strike (do not slap your feet to the ground).
- Allow your arms to swing freely from side to side.

The Foot and Walking Posture

The first part of walking begins with your foot touching the ground. The foot has two simple goals: making heel contact with the ground and making forefoot contact with the ground.

Goal #1: Heel contact with the ground

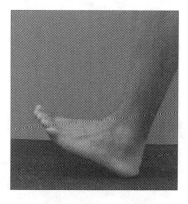

Goal #2: Forefoot contact with the ground

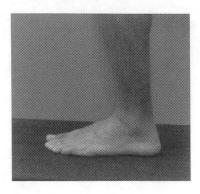

You may not realize it, but a lot goes on in your feet during a simple step. In order to properly contact the ground while absorbing forces and propelling you forward, your foot must change back and forth from a rigid lever into a mobile shock absorber. When your heel first strikes the ground, your foot is stable and rigid. Once the midfoot begins to make contact with the ground, your foot conforms to the ground surface and absorbs your body weight. Once all of your weight is accepted and absorbed, your foot changes back into a rigid lever propelling your body forward once the opposite heel makes contact with the ground. This rigidness allows the foot to push off the ground and propel your body forward without structural compromise or overstretching of your foot's tissue structures. Now let's take a look at what's happening to the rest of your body as you walk.

How Our Bodies Absorb Shock during Ambulation

As you walk, a large amount of force is placed on the muscles, from the foot, which first contacts the ground, all the way up to the upper cervical spine. The foot does its job by absorbing the force as it pronates and becomes a mobile adapter. But where does all this force go? As the foot absorbs the ground forces, these forces must be dissipated somewhere. If the force were to stop at the foot alone, there would be massive breakdown in that area.

A tour of the human body will help to make clear how force is distributed. As your heel strikes the ground and rolls forward, weight is accepted throughout your step at 120 percent of your body weight. This means that if a two-hundred-pound man is walking, every step he takes will put 240 pounds of pressure on his foot. This force is absorbed up the lower extremity. The majority of the force is transferred up the shin bone (tibia) and muscles to the knee, leaving about 15 percent of the force to be absorbed by the bone and muscles of the fibula, the bone located on the outside of the shin. From the knee, force is transferred up through the hip bone and muscles to the lower spine. Once the force has reached the lower spine, the thoracic spine, leading up to the cervical spine, accepts the rest of the force.

The amount of force that actually reaches all the way up to the neck depends on how good a job the muscles and tissues absorb the ground force. That's why it is important to have strong and well-positioned muscle length throughout the body.

If muscles are not strong enough to absorb the force, the bones and joints will have to. This will add unnecessary stress to the joints and in time may cause arthritis and joint pain.

Common Problem Areas

I have seen many patients with weakness in the external rotator of the hip. These rotators are deep muscles that travel from the front of the hips to the back of the hips and help stabilize the rotation of the knees. Someone with weak external hip rotators may experience knee pain because the knee is not efficiently being stabilized. When you land on your heel and weight is accepted through the lower extremity, your hip external rotators stabilize your hip as well as your knee joint by preventing internal hip rotation. When weight is accepted with weak hip external rotators, the muscles are not strong enough to stabilize the hip joint. Because of this the hip will rotate inward. This will rotate the knee inward (remember, the hip and knee are connected). Once this occurs, the force from the ground will put additional pressure on the inner aspect of the knee causing medial (inner) knee pain. With strong hip external rotator muscles, the knee is stabilized during weight acceptance, and force is distributed evenly throughout the lower extremities.

One way to demonstrate this concept is to first stand up and then let your knee buckle inward. Do you feel your hip muscles giving out?

Those are your external rotators, which, as discussed, are important for maintaining proper weight acceptance throughout your knee.

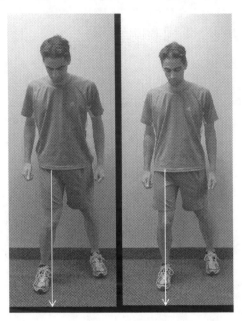

Proper Bending and Lifting

I have had many patients say, "I was just bending down, and I ended up hurting my back," or "My back hurts because I twisted wrong." Have you ever bent down too quickly and then wished you hadn't? Many people suffer from muscle strains because they don't use proper body mechanics while bending and lifting objects from the ground. Add muscle imbalance to the mix, and you are asking for an injury. Bending is one of the scariest things to do after a lower back injury. When my patients ask me how to bend, I tell them that the secret to bending properly is to think about it before doing it. This may be difficult for those who bend all day for a living but that is why it is important to train yourself beforehand so that when you aren't consciously thinking about it, you will subconsciously be doing it right. We must recognize the forces that are at play when we bend down to pick objects up from the floor. If you were to pick a spot on your lower spine and bend down using only your back, the force produced on the spine would be three times the force produced compared to bending with your knees.

Proper lifting properly disperses that weight throughout the body, which allows for a clean, pain-free lift. An added benefit to lifting properly is that it is a great way to improve hip external rotator muscle strength and essentially strengthen all of the body's major muscle groups. By bending properly, you reinforce, reeducate, and restrengthen your muscles!

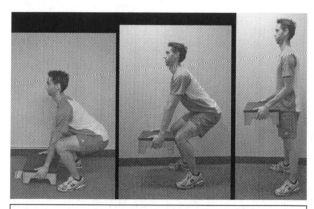

Proper lifting technique:
50-pound object = 50 pounds of force distributed
through the body

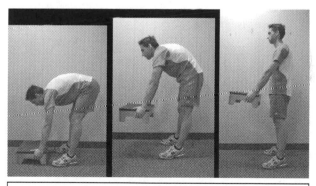

Improper lifting technique:
50-pound object × 3 = 150 pounds force directly on
the lower spine

Let's take a look at the correct picture and break this scenario down into simple steps.

The Descent

1. *Establish a solid base of support.* In order to use the least effort possible and reduce the risk of injury, we must first have a solid base of support. You accomplish this by keeping your feet flat, slightly pointed out, and shoulder-width apart, thus making your body more stable and well balanced.

NOTE: (Steps 2 and 3 performed simultaneously)

2. *Stick out your rear end.* Stick out your rear, as if you were sitting down on a chair. This will help your anatomical framework to withstand any forces placed upon the spine during the actual lift, thus preventing injury.

3. *Bend your knees.* Lower yourself by bending your knees. This will insure lower back safety. Do not let your knees buckle inward; keep them facing straight ahead. Remember, the body is made for your knees to withstand tremendous pressure. That's why we have 135 degrees of knee flexion available to us and only 60 degrees in the lower back.

4. *Keep your trunk parallel to your shins.* Keeping your trunk parallel to your shins will insure the spine is constantly in a stabilized position, which will help prevent unwanted back pain and injury.

5. *Keep the load close to your body.* While lifting, you want to keep the load as close to you as possible. This will immensely decrease the amount of work you need to perform to lift the object. Remember our discussion about holding a gallon of milk close to your body as opposed to further away? Just try it for yourself and feel the difference.

    Hold a gallon of milk in one hand with an outstretched arm for about ten seconds. Now bring the same gallon of milk close to your body and hold it for another ten seconds. Which task is easier?

6. *Keep weight in your heel arches.* When descending, make sure all of your weight is positioned through the heel arch of your feet. That is the part of your foot between your heel and foot arch. Your heels and your toes should not rise during a squat.

7. *Keep your collarbones up and out.* Making your upper extremity solid during a squat will prevent unwanted movements and thus prevent injury.

The Rise

Follow the same rules while rising with an object. Make sure you push up with your leg muscles and keep all of your weight centralized in the heel arch.

When lifting, remember these points:

1. Keep your eyes pointed straight ahead. If your eyes are pointed down, you are more likely to put additional strain on your upper neck.
2. Do not twist or turn as you lift. Rotatory forces are infamous for causing muscle strains in the lower back and rib areas.
3. Do not bend at the back.
4. If you are unable to keep the proper squat position while bending down or lifting an object, do not lift it. First, practice the technique as well as stretching and strengthening your muscles. Lift the object only after you are able to squat properly.

The Benefit of a Proper Squat

Above I mentioned that a proper squat will add additional strength to your muscles. I want to quickly touch upon this in a little more detail. By performing a proper squat, as described above, you are exercising essentially every major muscle in your body in one movement. Bending your knees strengthens your lower legs, quadriceps (front leg muscles), and hamstrings (back leg muscles), as well as your gluteal muscles (the muscles in your rear end) and hip external rotators (deep side hip muscles). By keeping your back straight while performing the squat, you strengthen the lower, mid, and upper back muscles as well as your core stomach muscles. Of course, lifting will also strengthen your arm muscles. In addition, by adopting proper form, you strengthen each muscle through its full range of motion. It is important not only to strengthen each muscle in the optimal position, but also through its full range of motion.

Chapter Five

The Importance of Proper Footwear

Proper footwear is very important. Just think about how much you walk in a given day, week, month, and year. Proper footwear plays a major role in absorbing shock and protecting your feet from injury. Shoes that fit poorly can lead to specific foot injuries, including but not limited to plantar fasciitis, ankle sprains, bunions, and hammertoes. In addition to local foot dysfunctions, improper footwear can cause dysfunctions at the ankle, knee, and above.

Many of my patients have come into my clinic with complaints of ankle, knee, hip, and lower back pain, all associated with improper footwear. Believe it or not, people can even acquire neck injuries from improper footwear! When you think about it, it makes sense. Your shoes and sneakers help your feet absorb shock and stabilize your body against ground reaction forces (see the discussion of dynamic movements in chapter 3). With each step taken, your foot absorbs all of your body weight and then propels your weight forward. Even if your shoes are not up to par, you still need to walk. Instead of your shoes absorbing and stabilizing the shock, your feet end up doing the job. And after our twenty thousandth step of the day, your feet may get a little fatigued. Depending on how well your muscles absorb the forces, they may continue up the chain to your knee, hip, and lower back, and up your spine to your neck. So be kind to your body and take a minute to learn about what makes a good shoe.

Shoe Design

The descriptions of the parts of a shoe below will give you a better idea of how your shoes protect your feet.

Heel

The heel absorbs most of the person's weight. The heel should have a broad base and be no higher than 4 centimeters. A higher heel will allow the shoe to absorb shock better and reduce strain, but it will decrease stability. You want to ensure that you have the proper combination of stability and shock absorption.

Heel Counter

This is the portion of the shoe that grasps the heel at the sides and back, preventing your heel from sliding up and down while you walk. The heel counter should be rigid and durable in order to stabilize your heel when your shoe contacts the ground.

Upper

This is the material that covers the top of the foot and composes the main part of the shoe. Dress shoes usually have leather uppers while sports shoes have synthetic fabric uppers, which tend to be lighter and breathe better.

Midsole

The midsole is located between the tread and the upper. The midsole controls excessive foot motion and provides cushioning and shock absorption.

Two common types of materials used in midsoles are EVA (ethylene vinyl acetate) and PU (polyurethane). EVA, a foam that is light and offers good cushioning, is most common, although the material does break down quickly. Compression-molded EVA is harder and more durable. PU, another type of foam, is more dense, heavy, and durable than EVA.

Outsole

This is the treaded layer glued to the bottom of the midsole. It resists wear, provides traction, and absorbs shock. The outsole is usually made of leather in dress shoes and rubber in athletic shoes.

Inner Sole

The inner sole is the inside of the shoe; it should be smooth and without seams, as excessive seams can lead to blisters and calluses.

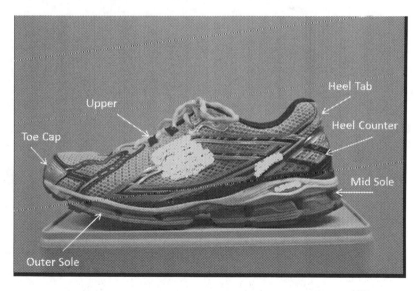

Proper Shoe Fit

Since we are on our feet for a big part of the day, it is very important to have a comfortable, fitting shoe. You can have the strongest, most durable, most shock-absorbent shoe on the market, but if it does not fit correctly, it won't do you any good. You need a shoe that feels good.

Before buying a pair of shoes, ask yourself what the purpose of the shoes is. Are they dress shoes, running shoes, or casual shoes? Then you want to find someone to fit you—someone who knows what they're talking about.

Keep these points in mind when choosing your shoes:

- Shoe size may vary among different shoe brands and styles so don't choose your shoes solely on size. Find the size you usually are, try it on, and then determine if it is the shoe you want.
- Try to choose a shoe that matches your foot. There are some shoes that have a higher arch for people with high arches, and shoes with lower arches to accommodate those with lower arches. In the end, it's all about comfort.
- Have your feet measured before trying on a shoe because your feet change as you grow older.
- It is better to try shoes on at the end of the day because by then you have walked around and your feet may have swelled since the morning. It's not fun to put on a shoe and realize by the end of the day that it is too tight. Shoes are made of strong material, and you should not expect them to stretch out to fit.
- If you are like most people, your feet are not the exact same size, so you should fit the shoe to your larger foot.
- Stand during the fitting process and check that there is adequate space (3/8 inch to ½ inch) for your longest toe at the end of each shoe. Make sure that the ball of your foot fits comfortably into the widest part (ball pocket) of the shoe and that there is minimal slippage in the heel.

Determining When to Buy a New Shoe

You may be wondering when you should get a new pair of shoes. Read on and determine what factors will alert you that you should buy a new pair of shoes.

Shoe Age

In order to determine whether or not your shoes are still adequate, you must first determine the age of your shoe. If you have owned a shoe for more than six months and you use them regularly, it is time to think about buying another pair. By then the shoe will have broken down and lost its ability to absorb shock and properly stabilize your foot. Runners need to replace their shoes every three months or every five hundred miles due to the excessive compression.

Shoe Inspection

Another way to determine when to buy new shoes is to look at the soles and the inside of your shoe. Check to see whether the shoe is worn and whether the treads are faded. If they are worn or faded, get rid of them; these shoes no longer serve their intended purpose of protecting your feet.

Outsole: Observe and determine whether the treads are worn/faded

Midsole: Compression Test: Press into the midsole of the shoe. The midsole should give and compress into your fingers. As the midsole wears down, it will not have as much give. When the midsole becomes stiff and shows creases or compression lines, it is time to replace your shoes.

Inner shoe: Observe whether the shoe has formed to your foot. If your shoe is stretched out you may acquire blisters in areas where you have not had them in the past.

Foot Injury Prevention

It is sometimes easy to prevent injury; this may be as simple as changing the type of shoe that you are wearing.

Sandals: During the summer months it is always fun to wear sandals because of their light weight and aesthetic features. Be aware, though, that sandals do cause foot problems. They offer very little shock absorption, minimal stability, and little protection from outside forces. If you have been wearing sandals for a while and complain of foot pain, decrease how often you wear sandals and consider wearing more durable shoes such as sneakers. This is an easy way to prevent further and more complicated problems. Sandals are known to damage the foot arches, which are the supporting structures of your feet.

In addition wearing sandals can increase muscle fatigue, thus preventing muscles from absorbing ground reaction forces and causing those forces to impact the joints and send pain up the chain.

High Heels: High heels place great unnatural stresses on the foot. Although viewed as aesthetically charming shoes in society, they are too narrow and too short. This can compress your toes together, which may cause problems such as hammertoes and bunions. Also, when you walk in high heels, your calf muscles are placed in a shortened position. This causes the calf muscle fibers and Achilles tendon to shorten and become tight, which in turn will cause the ankle to lose motion. The loss of motion and tight musculature can lead to calf strains, Achilles tendonitis, and other related foot problems.

Chapter Six

Muscle Matters: Stretching and Strengthening

Stretching your muscles is very important in maintaining proper, pain-free posture. If your muscles are stretched to their normal length, they will be better able to stabilize and hold you in the correct position. If your muscles are shortened, they will pull on your joints, preventing movement and placing them in a position more prone for injury. Strengthening the muscle is just as important in maintaining proper posture. If your muscles are strong, they will hold you in the correct static position longer and will allow you to move more efficiently for longer periods of time. Our goal is to keep our muscles strong and at their optimal lengths through stretching and strengthening. If your muscles are stronger and properly stretched, they will have more strength and endurance, allowing greater static and dynamic postural stabilization.

Four Main Stretches

1. Dynamic stretch
2. Static stretch
3. Ballistic stretch
4. Peripheral neuromuscular facilitation (PNF) stretch

For our purposes, we will focus on the static and dynamic stretches. Although I have included a brief description of ballistic and PNF stretches, I do not advise you perform these two stretches since greater injury can occur if they are performed incorrectly.

Dynamic Stretch

A dynamic stretch uses speed of movement, momentum, and active muscular effort to bring about a stretch. Unlike static stretching, the end position is not held. You should engage in dynamic stretching before beginning any sport activity and before doing any static stretching; it is important to get your blood moving in order to warm up your muscles before holding a static stretch. A ten-minute warm up consisting of dynamic stretching is optimal in order to raise your heart rate and increase blood flow. If you do not have that much time, take at least a few minutes to perform dynamic stretching before moving on to your static stretches. The picture below demonstrates a walking lunge.

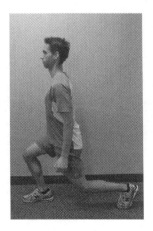

Static Stretch

A static stretch is a stretch that is performed and held for a given amount of time. You never want to stretch a "cold" muscle. This will increase your chances of straining or pulling that muscle, which can result in injury. A static stretch is best performed after warm-up exercises and after dynamic stretching. This is especially important if you plan to engage in any sport activity afterward.

Through scientific research, the healthcare field has determined that a static stretch held for a time period of thirty to sixty seconds is optimal for muscle elongation. Stretches should be performed for three to four sets for at least a thirty-second hold before and after exercise.

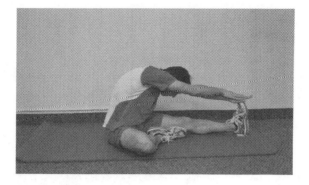

Ballistic Stretch

Ballistic stretching involves active muscular movement at end range. It is a combination of the static and dynamic stretch that uses a bouncing and jerking motion to increase muscle length and range of motion. The ballistic stretch requires caution and care. Due to the bouncing, people who perform these stretches are at greater risk of straining their muscles. If you have had a recent injury (up to six weeks prior), I would not recommend this type of stretch. I also do not recommend even trying this stretch unless you have had a personal trainer or physical therapist demonstrate the proper technique and observe you engage in the stretch.

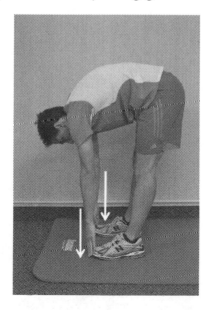

Peripheral Neuromuscular Facilitation (PNF)

PNF stretching was originally developed as a form of rehabilitation. It is a very effective stretching technique that requires a partner in order for it to be performed correctly. Although PNF is an effective form of stretching, certain precautions need to be taken, as PNF stretching can put added stress on the targeted muscle group, which can increase the risk of soft tissue injury.

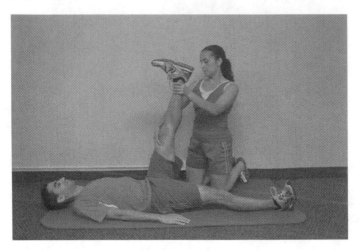

The Three Muscle Actions

Muscle can be either lengthened or shortened through movement. When a muscle is relaxed, it is in a preferred neutral state.

There are three basic muscle actions:

1. Concentric muscle action
2. Eccentric muscle action
3. Isometric muscle action

Concentric Muscle Action

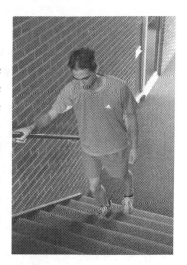

During a concentric muscle action, the muscle shortens because the contractile force is greater than the resistive force. The force generated within the muscle that is acting to shorten it is stronger than the resistive force that is acting on the tendons to stretch it.

When you are walking up stairs, your quadriceps muscles are generating more force than the resistive force of gravity, allowing you to advance your body upward.

Eccentric Muscle Action

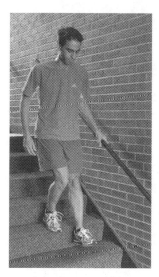

An eccentric muscle action is one in which the muscle lengthens because the contractile force is less than the resistive forces. The force that is acting to shorten the muscle is weaker than the force acting on the tendons to stretch it. Eccentric muscle action controls movement. While you are going down stairs, the quadriceps muscles of your weight-bearing leg are downwardly controlling your body movement by preventing your foot from slamming to the ground with each step. Also when you are performing resistance training or lifting weights, the eccentric muscle action prevents the weight from being accelerated downward by gravity.

Isometric Muscle Action

An isometric muscle action is one in which the muscle length does not change because the contractile force is equal to the resistive force. The forces acting to shorten a muscle are equal to the resistive forces acting to lengthen it. In other words, we are exerting force but we are not moving. Isometric control is used to stay in a proper posture.

Because the resistive force of gravity is always pulling down on us, our postural stabilizing muscles must work to equal that amount of force to keep us static and controlled.

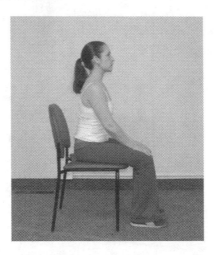

Tight Muscle versus Strong Muscle

Do not be confused between the two terms tight and strong. These are very different from one another. A tight muscle feels hard just like a strong muscle does, but unlike strong muscle, it is not at its proper length. Someone with forward head posture will have tight front neck musculature; the neck may feel strong to touch, but that tightness is detrimental to the overall positioning of the neck and head. Strong front neck muscles will place the head and neck in the proper position and hold it there safely. The same thing applies for someone who has tight hamstring muscles. The muscles will feel hard in the back of the leg, but if you ask the person to squat, he or she will have difficulty holding the proper position because the back leg muscles will be at an improper length and will not have the adequate range of motion to move the body through that proper functional motion.

That is why a combination of stretching and strengthening through one's full range of motion is key in maintaining the muscle at its proper length. A tight muscle can lead to muscle strains and injury.

When Acute Pain Strikes

When acute neck or back pain begins, taking certain measures will increase your odds of recovering more quickly and more efficiently. First, you want to be aware of and maintain proper posture as described in chapters two and three. Then you should perform the postural exercises described in this book. If pain persists, put some ice on the muscle for about ten to fifteen minutes. Icing for less than ten minutes will not provide the full therapeutic effect, and applying ice for more than fifteen minutes will put you at a greater risk for developing skin irritation. Ice helps calm the injured area and decrease blood flow. A useful acronym that I give to my patients is *RICE*:

- *Rest*: Rest the injured area. It is important to rest in order for the body to heal itself.
- *Ice*: Ice the sore area for at least ten minutes. Make sure to put a layer (e.g., a pillow case, a towel, or some other cloth) between the ice pack and your skin in order to prevent skin irritation.
- *Compression*: Compress the injured site while icing. This will help decrease inflammation.
- *Elevation*: Elevate the injured site above your heart if it is any part of your lower extremity. This will allow the inflammatory fluids to be reabsorbed into the lymph system via the heart and then be disposed of through urine.

Once acute pain has ended, at least one week after injury, and when your muscles feel more tight then painful, heat the injured area. You can buy microwavable heat packs that provide moist heat after they are microwaved. Electric blankets and heating pads are also beneficial. Just remember to turn them off and try not to fall asleep with them on. Too much heat can cause burns. Hot showers and baths are also beneficial. I recommend not performing stretches in the shower, although it may be tempting to do so, because you can easily slip and pull a muscle, or fall and cause further, more serious injury.

If you are going to soak in the bath make sure you do not prop your head up against the tub; that will push your neck forward, causing excessive forward neck posture. If your tub is not large enough for you to place your neck in the proper postural position while you are soaking, please consider using another method of heat. Do not perform activities that put your head in a forward flexed position, such as reading a book or performing computer work. This will put additional stress on the already damaged tissues and muscles.

Gauging Your Discomfort During Exercise

In preparation for the exercise protocol section I wanted to review when and when not to push through pain. Many patients ask me, "At what point do I stop exercising if I experience pain?" It is safe to say that one should stop exercising if the discomfort becomes worse than a five out of ten on a zero-to-ten pain scale, where zero is no pain, and ten is severe pain requiring hospitalization.

Another useful way to gauge whether you can safely continue exercising is to use the red/yellow/green-light method. If your discomfort is getting better with exercise, then you have the green light to continue performing your exercise. If the exercise does not change your discomfort, then you have a yellow light to proceed with caution—but be aware of your body's response. If you perform an exercise and it causes increased pain and discomfort, this is a red light to stop. As you continue to perform the exercise, ask yourself, "Is my discomfort feeling the same, is it getting better, or is it getting worse?"

By following the red/yellow/green-light method and being aware of your symptoms, you can safely and effectively perform exercises without the worry of causing additional harm to your body.

Now that you understand why posture is important, and you know the proper way to sit, stand, walk, and squat, you are ready to further explore how to condition your body to make this all possible. Because you have been in your former posture for so long you must now undo your muscular imbalances. In order to improve upon these muscle imbalances, you must stretch and strengthen your muscles to their appropriate lengths so that they are better able to stabilize your spine and perform their given functions. The next part of this book will guide you through specific exercise protocols that will help you perform static and dynamic activities safely and effectively. So let's get to it!

Chapter Seven

Two-Step Stretch and Strengthening Protocols

I have compiled a two-step process to successfully rebuild proper posture. The first-step protocol consists of basic dynamic and static stretches combined with basic strengthening exercises geared toward improving muscular range of motion and muscular proprioception. The second-step protocol consists of dynamic strengthening and utilization of core musculature to produce what I call "strong motion." I define strong motion as muscular stability throughout a full range of motion.

First-Step protocol

I have provided three basic protocols that will provide the body with adequate warm-up, range of motion, and muscle awareness to withstand normal daily stressors that require mild to moderate physical exertion. These protocols will build a framework that allows the body to maintain proper postural control during sitting, standing, walking, and bending.

- Five-Minute Dynamic Stretch Protocol
- Ten-Minute Static Stretch Protocol
- Ten-Minute Strengthening Protocol

Second-Step protocol

The next two protocols are the second step in the process that will build upon the first three protocols. The dynamic structural strengthening protocol, combined with core stabilization protocol, will provide the body with the strong motion needed to perform proper lifting technique and to play sports of mild to moderate intensity with a decreased chance of muscular injury.

- Ten-Minute Dynamic Structural Strengthening Protocol
- Ten-Minute Core Stabilization Protocol

Five-Minute Dynamic Stretching Protocol

The dynamic stretching protocol provides the necessary movements needed to safely and efficiently warm up our body prior to engaging in static stretching exercises. With these movements you will increase your functional range of motion and decrease the risk of muscle pulls.

1. Neck mobility (flexion, extension, lateral flexion, rotation)
2. Shoulder shrugs
3. Arm swings
4. Hip circles and twists
5. Standing marching

Neck Mobility

Warm-up neck exercises are important to perform in the morning in order to loosen up your muscles and allow them to acclimate to movement after they have been static for many hours during the night. It is also important to perform them throughout the day if you sit at a desk for many hours.

Neck Flexion and Extension

Begin by slowly tucking your chin down toward your chest. Slowly lift your chin up until you have extended your neck as far back as you comfortably can go. Perform this exercise ten to fifteen times in each direction or until you feel less restricted in this particular motion.

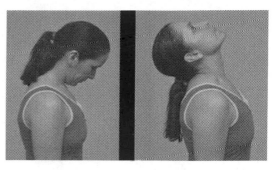

Neck Lateral Flexion

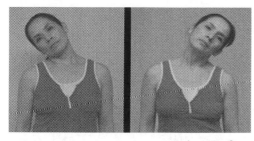

Begin by gently lowering your left ear toward your left shoulder and then returning your head position to neutral. Next, gently lower your right ear toward your right shoulder. Be sure not to lift your shoulder to your ear—a common mistake. Perform this exercise ten to fifteen times on each side or until your motion feels fluid and effortless.

Neck Rotation

Begin by gently turning your chin toward your left shoulder. Return to neutral (face forward), and then gently turn your chin toward your right shoulder. Perform this exercise ten to fifteen times on each side or until this motion becomes easy to perform.

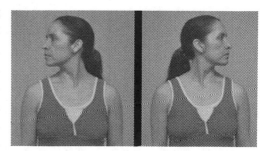

Forward and Backward Shoulder Shrugs

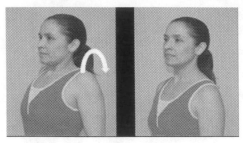

Shoulder shrugs help loosen up your shoulders and upper spine.

Begin by standing in proper posture. Raise both shoulders up toward your ears and slowly push your shoulders toward the front of your body in a circular motion. Perform this exercise twenty to thirty times or until your shoulders begin to feel loose.

Next, raise both shoulders up toward your ears and back, slowly pulling your shoulder blades down in a circular motion. Perform this exercise twenty to thirty times or until your shoulder begins to feel loose.

Arm Swings

Arm swings are helpful in loosening up your shoulders and warming up your upper extremity.

Begin by standing in a proper posture. Raise both arms out to the side, keeping them at shoulder height. Slowly and gently move your arms in a circular motion starting off small and increasing the circumference of the circles as you go. Perform this exercise in a forward direction twenty times or until your arms begin to feel loose. Then perform the reverse motion twenty times or until your arms feel loose.

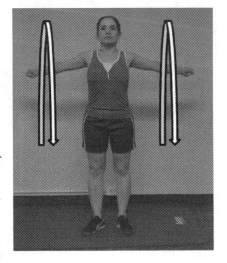

Hip Circles

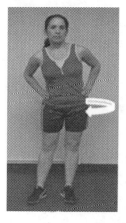

Hip circles loosen up your hips and lower back without putting excessive strain on your back musculature.

Begin by standing with your hands on your hips and your feet spread slightly wider than shoulder width. Slowly and gently make circles with your hips in a clockwise direction twenty times. Then repeat the similar motion in a counterclockwise direction another twenty times. You should feel your core and midsection loosen up.

Hip Twists

Hip twists also loosen up the hip and lower back muscles without putting excessive strain on the muscles of the back.

Begin by standing with your hands on your side with your feet spread slightly wider than shoulder width. Twist your torso and hips to the right while at the same time shifting your weight onto the left foot. Then twist your torso and hips to the left while shifting your weight to the right foot. Perform this exercise twenty times on each side, or until you feel loose in the hips.

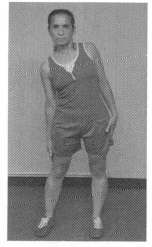

Standing Marching

Standing marching helps warm up and loosen up the lower extremity, including the hips, knees, and ankles. Standing in your proper posture, begin to march in place bringing your knees up as high as comfortably possible. Repeat this motion twenty times or until your lower extremity becomes loose.

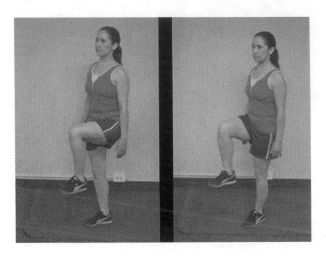

Five-Minute Dynamic Stretching Protocol

Exercise	Sets and Reps	Frequency	Modifications
Neck flexion	10 to 15 times each direction	2 times per day	N/A
Neck extension	10 to15 times in each direction	2 times per day	N/A
Neck lateral flexion	10 to15 times in each direction	2 times per day	N/A
Rotation	10 to15 times in each direction	2 times per day	N/A
Shoulder shrugs	2 to 3 sets of 10	2 times per day	N/A
Arm swing	20 times	2 times per day	N/A
Hip circles	20 times	2 times per day	N/A
Hip twists	20 times	2 times per day	N/A
Standing marching	3 sets of 10	2 times per day	N/A

Ten-Minute Static Stretching Protocol

By performing this protocol you will improve flexibility in your back and lower limbs, which will allow you to maintain a better posture in sitting, standing, and bending technique.

1. Thera Ball midback stretch
2. Sitting thoracic mobilizations
3. Press-ups
4. Standing back extensions
5. Hamstring stretch (choose one)
   a. Standing
   b. Sitting
   c. Lying

6. Doorway stretch
7. Corner Stretch
8. Quadriceps stretch

Thera Ball Midback Stretch

This exercise is ideal for stretching out the thoracic spine, an area that is commonly tight, which can affect many joints of the body up and down the functional chain. Remember, a tight midback will prevent you from keeping your chest up and out while sitting, and standing, and will keep you from achieving the desired parallel chest-to-shin stature during a squat technique.

Lean back on a Thera Ball and hold your position for one minute. If you are still comfortable, try to hold the position for another minute or so. Once your back loosens up, you will be able to hold this position for an even longer length of time. I would recommend working your way up to holding the position for about three minutes.

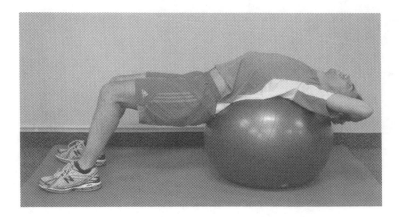

Sitting Thoracic Mobilization

Begin by sitting with your back against a chair. Slowly bend back so that the upper mid back is being pushed into the top of the back of the chair. This will help loosen your thoracic spine. Perform this mobilization ten to twenty times or until your midback feels loose.

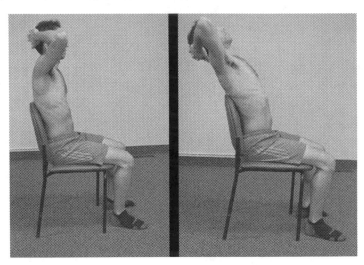

Press-Ups

This exercise will increase motion in your lower back by loosening up the vertebral joints. This exercise is also discussed earlier in the book.

Lying prone on your stomach, perform a press-up by

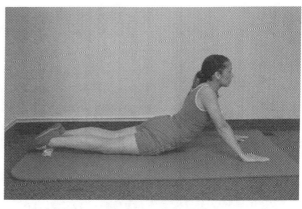

bringing your hands close to your chest, shoulder-width apart and with elbows bent. Press your hands into the floor lifting your trunk up while at the same time keeping your lower body on the ground.

Standing Back Extension

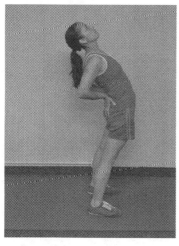

This is an adaptation of the prone press-up exercise and can more feasibly be performed while you are at work. While standing, place your hands behind your back and slowly tilt your back as far as possible. Once you have reached your end range of motion, slowly return to a neutral standing position. Try not to bend your knees or move your hips. Perform this exercise twenty to thirty times or until you feel your lower back loosen up. To target specific segments of your spine, place your hands on both sides of the targeted vertebrae and bend back.

It is important to note that if this exercise causes irritation to your lower back, the prone press-up exercise may be more suitable to perform while starting out. Less stress is placed on the vertebral joints in the prone position.

Hamstring Stretches

There are many ways to stretch the hamstrings. The hamstrings are important muscles to keep limber because they have attachments to the hips that are directly related to motion and flexibility of the spine. They also reinforce proper walking and bending technique. You want to have about 90 degrees of pure passive hamstring motion. Too much can provide excessive movement, which may lead to negative hip and lower back issues if your muscles are not strong enough at those end ranges. I will review a few stretches that I have found to be most beneficial to my patients.

Standing Hamstring Stretch

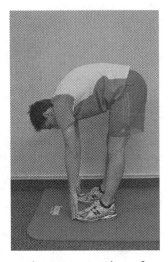

The standing hamstring stretch is an easy-to-perform stretch that can be done just about anywhere. In stretches not only the hamstring muscle but also the gluteal muscles as well as the small lower and midback muscles known as the erector spinae group.

Start in a standing position with your feet about six inches apart from one another. Slowly bend down with your arms outstretched and attempt to touch your toes. If you are unable to touch your toes, go as far as you can until you feel a mild stretch. If you want to target the inner hamstring muscles, perform the same exercise, but this time spread your feet apart about two to three feet while pointing your toes out.

Hamstring Towel Stretch

The hamstring towel stretch allows your lower extremity muscles to relax while you are stretching. You don't need to fire your front quad and hip flexor muscles as you do to bend in the first hamstring stretch.

Lie down on your back and bend your nonstretching leg to about 45 degrees. This will prevent back pain during the exercise. Wrap a towel around the foot of the leg you will be stretching. With that leg straight, pull up on the towel and slowly raise your leg as high as you can to the point where you feel a comfortable stretch with only mild to moderate discomfort. Perform four times, holding for thirty seconds each time. (Note: You can substitute a dog leash, belt, jump rope, or the like for a towel.)

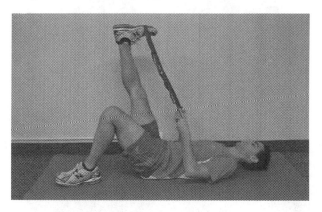

Sitting Hamstring Stretch

The sitting hamstring stretch is a nice stretch to perform because in addition to stretching your hamstrings, you target necessary lower back musculature such as the erector spinae group and the quadratus lumborum.

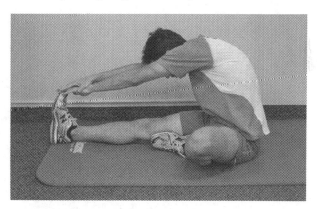

Sit on the floor with your legs pointed straight ahead. Keep the stretching leg straight and bend the nonstretching leg toward your groin so that the bottom of your foot is against the inner thigh of the stretching leg. Once in this position, gently lean forward with one hand outstretched over the other and reach for your toes. Stretch only to the point where you feel a mild to moderate stretch. Do this four times, holding for thirty seconds each time.

Note: If this stretch aggravates your back you can use a towel to pull your foot toward you rather than bending forward. This stretch will not target your lower back muscles.

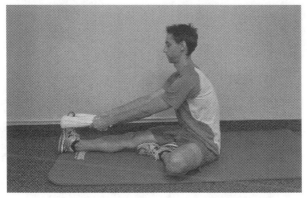

Substitution: Sitting towel Stretch

Doorway Stretch

I enjoy this stretch because it targets the infamous tight pectoral muscles that are common to many people who slouch in their chairs throughout the day. In addition to stretching the front chest musculature, this stretch also places the shoulder blades in their proper anatomical position, reminding the body of where they should be.

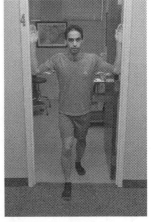

Find a doorway narrow enough to allow you to place both forearms against the sides of the wall. Place both forearms against the wall at about shoulder height. Advance one leg through the doorway and bend the knee. Lean into the stretch and put some weight onto the bent knee. You want to feel mild discomfort at most during any stretch. Complete the stretch four times, holding for thirty to sixty seconds each time.

Corner Stretch

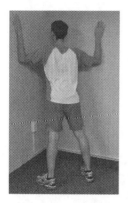

If the doorways are just too wide for your arms, you can try the corner stretch instead. Though I find that the corner stretch is not as effective, it is better than nothing and will stretch your front musculature nonetheless.

Stand in a corner with your hands raised to shoulder level. Lean forward until you feel a comfortable stretch across your chest. Complete the stretch four times, holding for thirty seconds each time.

Ten-Minute Static Stretching Protocol

Exercise	Sets and Reps	Frequency	Modifications
Thera Ball stretch	3 sets (1 minute ea.)	2 times per day	N/A
Sitting thoracic mobilizations	3 sets of 10	2 times per day	N/A
Press-ups	3 sets of 10	2 times per day	N/A
Standing back extension	3 sets of 10	2 times per day	N/A
Hamstring stretch	30 sec.; hold 4 times	2 times per day	Standing, sitting, lying
Doorway stretch	30 sec.; hold 4 times	2 times per day	N/A
Corner stretch	30 sec.; hold 4 times	2 times per day	N/A
Quadriceps stretch	30 sec.; hold 4 times	2 times per day	N/A

Ten-Minute Strengthening Protocol

The five exercises listed below will improve shoulder blade and midback posture.

1. Chin tucks
2. Shoulder blade squeezes
3. Opposite arm and leg
4. Standing hip extension
5. Quadruped hip abduction (fire hydrants)

Chin tucks

This exercise prevents forward head posture and helps strengthen the frontal neck muscles. (This exercise was also discussed in the forward head posture section of this book under four common postural deficits) While in a seated or standing position, adopt a proper posture with your chest up and out. Next, retract or tuck your head back. Be sure not to bend your chin or neck while performing this movement. It is strictly a backward movement.

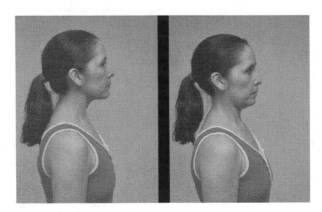

Shoulder Blade Squeezes

In a seated or standing position (depending on what posture you have more difficulty with) keep your arms by your side squeeze your shoulder blades together as if you were trying to hold a ball between your shoulder blades. (This 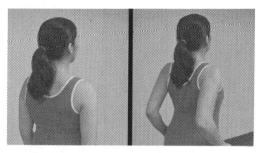 exercise was also discussed in the forward head posture section of this book under four common postural deficits)

Opposite Arm and Leg

This exercise is important because it targets the back muscles and core stomach muscles, which aid in stabilizing the trunk during standing and ambulation.

Start this exercise on your hands and knees. Raise one arm outstretched in front of you as you raise and straighten out the opposite leg. Complete this exercise five times on each side, holding the position for ten seconds each time.

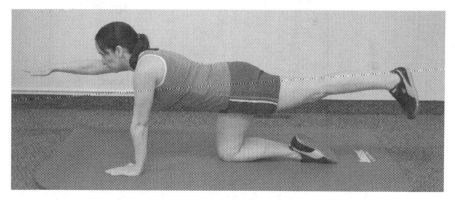

Standing Hip Extension

This exercise is helpful in strengthening the lower lumbar and gluteal muscles. Stand with proper posture. Slowly extend one leg about twelve inches back while stabilizing yourself on the opposite leg. Make sure that your posture is not jeopardized when performing the exercise. Holding on to a countertop for support is recommended.

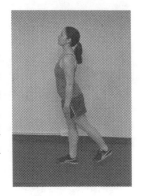

Quadruped Hip Abduction (Fire Hydrant)

This exercise helps strengthen the hip external rotators. Begin in a quadruped position (on hands and knees). Raise one leg out to the side with your knee bent, raising the knee up about two feet high. Slowly lower your leg down and perform this exercise for three sets of ten.

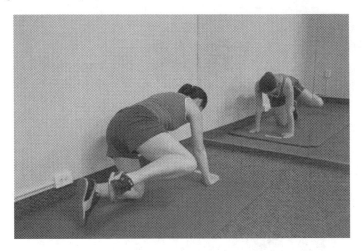

Ten-Minute Strengthening Protocol

Exercise	Sets and Reps	Frequency	Modifications
Chin tucks	3 sets of 10	2 times per day	Sitting, standing, lying on back
Shoulder blade squeezes	3 sets of 10	2 times per day	N/A
Opposite arm and leg	5 sets each side (hold for 10 sec.)	2 times per day	N/A
Standing hip extension	3 sets of 10	2 times per day	N/A
Quadruped hip abduction (fire hydrants)	3 sets of 10	2 times per day	N/A

Ten-Minute Core Strengthening Protocol

The core consists of the stomach musculature, lower back stabilizers, midback stabilizers, and hip musculature. A strong core is important because it helps stabilize the rest of your body while you are performing dynamic movements. The six exercises listed below will stabilize your core.

1. Posterior pelvic tilts
2. Planks
3. Side planks
4. Crunches
5. Prone back extension
6. Side-lying sweeps

Posterior Pelvic Tilt

A posterior pelvic tilt is a simple exercise that takes practice to perform correctly. It is not a very functional exercise, but to learn how to perform this exercise functionally, we need to begin with its simplest form and build up from there. First let's review a pelvic tilt.

Lie on your back and bend both knees so that your feet are comfortably resting on the floor. Keep both arms by your side in a relaxed position. Then slowly pull your belly button down to the floor using your stomach muscles so that the small of your back makes contact with the ground. Hold this position for ten seconds and repeat ten times.

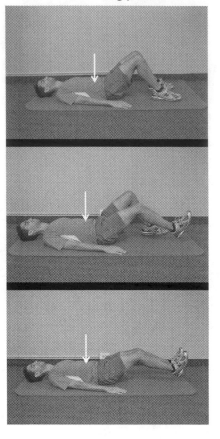

Functional Posterior Pelvic Tilt

Now that you can perform a pelvic tilt, it is important to incorporate this exercise into your daily routine in order to make it functional. When are we ever going to lie on our backs and tighten our stomach muscles? It is not a functional exercise, so let's make it so. Instead of performing a pelvic tilt while lying down, perform the exercise while sitting in a chair. You can also perform the exercise while standing against the wall. By placing yourself in positions that you sustain throughout the day, you make this exercise functional.

Planks

Planks help strengthen the center and side muscle groups of the stomach. There are two types of planks, the beginner plank and the full plank. The beginner plank requires less strength and should be performed first if you have never done a plank before.

Beginner Plank

Start by placing yourself in a quadruped position on all fours. Then come down on your forearms and on your knees. Your arms should be shoulder-width apart.

Keep your back straight and hold yourself in this position (aim to work your way up to holding the position for thirty seconds, four times). If you cannot hold for thirty seconds, that's okay. Work up to it by holding for ten and then twenty and eventually thirty seconds.

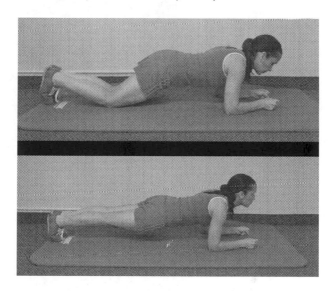

Full Plank

Begin by placing yourself in a quadruped position on all fours. Then come down on your forearms and on your toes. Your arms and feet should be shoulder-width apart. Keep your back straight and hold yourself in this position (aim to hold the position four times for thirty seconds each).

Side Planks

Start by lying on your right side. Prop yourself up on your right forearm. Then support yourself on your right foot with your left foot placed on top of the right. Keep your back straight. Hold for thirty seconds if possible and perform the exercise four times. Repeat this on the left side.

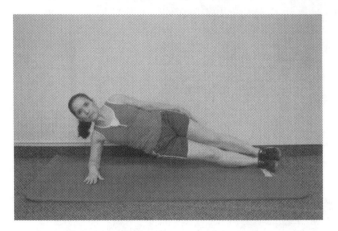

Crunch Progressions

The crunch exercise is a popular exercise to strengthen the rectus abdominis or "six pack" muscle. Listed below are three progressions which will challenge your muscles as you progress.

Crunch I

Lie on your back with your knees bent up to 45 degrees. Place your arms on the floor fully extended. Next, pull your chest toward your knees and raise your shoulder blades about four to six inches off the floor. Do not use your arms to help lift your trunk up. Hold for about one second and slowly control your descent back down. Perform three sets of ten.

Crunch II

Perform the crunch exercise described above but rather than extending your arms at your sides, fold them over each other, resting on your chest.

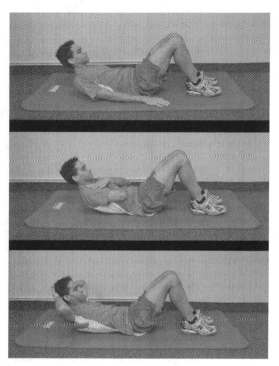

Crunch III

Perform the same crunch exercise with your arms behind your head and your hands interlocked. Make sure you do not use your arms to pull yourself up while performing the crunch. If you cannot perform a crunch without the help of your arms, go back to the crunch II exercise.

Prone Back Extension

Prone Press-Ups (Back Extension I):

While lying prone (on your stomach), keep your arms shoulder-width apart and use your arms to lightly push up your upper body. Use your lower back muscles to aid in the upward motion, keeping your hips and lower extremity on the floor. Hold for about five seconds and then slowly control your descent down with your arms and your lower back muscles. The less you push with your hands, the more your lower back muscles will work.

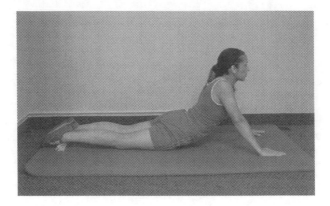

Prone Back (Back Extension II)

While lying prone, keep your arms at your side and perform the same back extension exercise without using your arms. Hold for about five seconds and slowly control your descent down. Perform ten times and then relax.

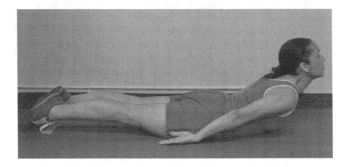

Side-Lying Sweeps

This exercise targets the external rotators, abductors, and extensors of your hips and is a very beneficial exercise to help strengthen them.

Start by lying on your side. Keep your body straight from your head to your toes. This exercise consists of three movements, which are performed simultaneously. The first movement is raising your leg up toward the ceiling, making sure that your knee is locked. For the second movement rotate your hip outward so that your toes point toward the ceiling. The third movement is slightly extending your hip or bringing your leg back.

Perform these three movements at the same time. Then bring your leg back to the side-lying position. Perform three sets of ten on each leg.

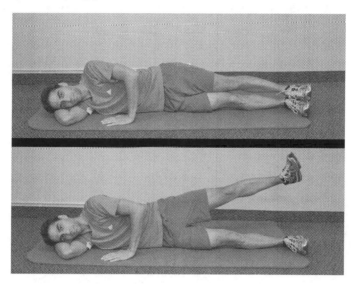

Ten-Minute Core-Strengthening Protocol

Exercise	Sets and Reps	Frequency	Modifications
Posterior pelvic tilt	3 sets of 10	2 times per day	While sitting or standing
Planks	3 sets of 10	2 times per day	On knees, on toes
Side planks	3 sets of 10	2 times per day	Arm pointed up
Crunches	3 sets of 10	2 times per day	Arms at side, arms folded in front, arms crossed behind head
Prone back extension	2 to 3 sets of 10	2 times per day	With press-up assist, arms at side
Side lying sweeps	2 to 3 sets of 10	2 times per day	N/A

Ten-Minute Dynamic Structural Strengthening Protocol

A structural exercise uses multiple joints throughout a single movement. This type of exercise targets the whole muscular chain instead of singling out specific muscles. Structural exercises are more advanced but at the same time more functional. Do not attempt to perform these until you have mastered the basic exercise protocols.

1. Walking lunges
2. Step-ups
3. Heel taps
4. Squats
5. Lateral side walk

Lunges

Lunges are a great exercise to strengthen the front thigh, hamstring, buttock, and side hip muscles. Since the body is kept erect throughout the movement, all core stabilizers work to prevent gravity from disrupting the proper posture.

Walking Lunge

With your body erect and your arms comfortably at your sides, take a step forward, landing on the heel arch of your foot (the area between the heel of your foot and the forefoot). Make sure that, when your lead foot (the foot in front) hits the ground, it stays down and your heel does not rise. Once you land on your lead foot, begin to lower yourself toward the ground by bending with both legs. Your back heel should come up on the back foot once you begin to lower yourself. Allow the knee of your back leg to lightly tap the ground. Once your knee touches the ground, raise yourself back up and alternate positions, allowing your back leg to become the lead leg. Repeat these steps, moving forward (i.e., across the room or down the hallway). Perform three sets of ten.

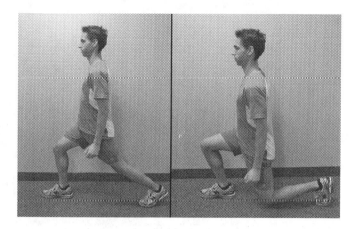

Walking Lunges with Weight Bar

With your body erect and a weight bar resting on the back of your shoulders, perform the walking lunge exercise described above. The addition of the bar will challenge your body more because of the extra weight.

Lunge with Snatch Grip

Stand up tall and hold the weight bar with a snatch grip. (A snatch grip is when you hold the bar about four inches over your head, making sure your elbows are locked out at all times.)

Make sure the bar always stays over your head. Try to avoid having the bar move back and forth, for it is easy to lose control throughout the exercise. Next, perform your lunge as described above. By lunging with your arms overhead, holding the weight bar with a snatch grip, you will target the upper extremity musculature along with the lower extremity musculature.

Step-Ups

This dynamic exercise improves quadriceps strength as well as gluteal, hamstring, hip flexor, and trunk strength. It is very functional, as it simulates the action of ascending stairs.

Step-Up

Start with a moderate step (six to eight inches) to begin with. A normal staircase step is eight inches high. Step up with your dominant foot, making sure that you land on the heel arch of your foot and push yourself up with that foot. Do not allow your grounded foot to help. Once 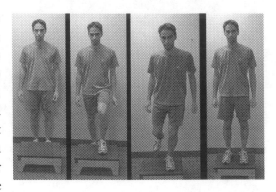 you have stepped up and placed your two feet on the step, step back down with your opposite foot first, allowing your dominant foot to control the descent and distributing the weight into the heel arch. Perform three sets of ten repetitions; then repeat this exercise using your nondominant leg.

Step-Up with Arm Raise

Perform the same step-up exercise, but this time, add an upward arm swing. Raise your arms above your head while you lift yourself up with your lead leg. When stepping down, swing your arms back down.

Lateral Step-Ups

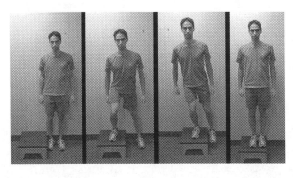

Lateral step-ups are good for strengthening side hip muscles.

Standing in an erect position, face to the side. Step up with your dominant foot landing on your heel arch. Use that foot to raise yourself up onto the step. Then slowly lower yourself down controlling your descent with your dominant foot.

Heel Taps

The heel tap is a functional exercise that simulates a stepping-down motion.

Using a step or stairs, slowly tap your leading heel to the ground by controlling your descent with the opposite leg. Make sure your weight is distributed into the heel arch of your stabilizing knee. Also be sure that your stabilizing knee does not bend inward and that your stabilizing hip does not collapse inward while your lead heel lightly taps the ground.

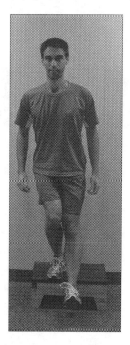

Squats

Start by standing with your feet shoulder-width apart with your toes slightly facing out to the side. Keep your arms by your side or hold onto a stick or weight bar as shown in the picture. Slowly bend your knees keeping your weight on the heel arches of both feet. As you descend make sure to keep your rear end out and your chest up so that the bending motion occurs in your knees, not at your waist. Rise by pushing through your heel arches, straightening your legs, and keeping your back straight. Complete three sets of ten repetitions. As you improve, you can add weight; in this protocol, though, we are focusing on functional postural correction, not strength training.

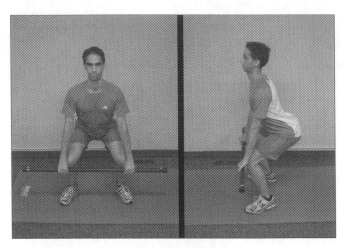

Lateral Side Walks

Start by getting into a half-squat position. Hold on to a stick and let it hang down to your knees loosely. Once in this position take a side step in one direction with one leg and then move the other leg in that same direction. Make sure your knees stay bent and your feet point forward. Do not drag your feet on the ground while stepping out to the side.

Keep stepping in one direction for about twenty steps. Then sidestep back to your starting point another twenty steps. This will help strengthen your quadriceps, external hip rotators, and side leg muscles. To make this exercise more challenging, you can wrap a Thera-Band around your legs.

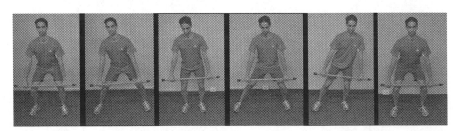

Ten-Minute Dynamic Structural Strengthening Protocol

Exercise	Sets and Reps	Frequency	Modifications
Walking Lunge	3 sets of 10	2 times per day	Weighted bar Snatch grip
Step ups	3 sets of 10	2 times per day	Arm raise during the rise
Side step ups	3 sets of 10	2 times per day	Arm raise during the rise
Heel Taps	2 to 3 sets of 10	2 times per day	N/A
Squats	2 to 3 sets of 10	2 times per day	Back squats with weight, snatch grip squats
Lateral Side Walk	20 to 30 steps in each direction	2 times per day	Weight in hands (no more than 20 lbs.)

Chapter Eight

When to Seek Professional Help

Though this book is intended to help you to self-correct and improve your posture, at times medical attention will be needed. This book covers the basics of postural correction and is not intended to resolve all dysfunctions. The following section includes information intended to help you know when to seek professional help.

There are four sensations that can help guide you in assessing the severity of your dysfunction. Aching pain is usually the first sensation you will feel after something is chronically disrupted or acutely disturbed within your body. Sharp pain is the next sensation that will come along. Tingling comes next, followed finally by numbness. With numbness, the nerve is being compressed so much that it is unable to accept signals from the brain in response to a stimulus such as touch. If you experience numbness, see your doctor or physical therapist, but do not panic. I have treated many patients with numbness and tingling. Once certain techniques are performed and patients have a good understanding of how to maintain proper posture, they turn out fine.

Earlier in the book, I briefly discussed how sitting incorrectly can cause pain, tingling, or numbness travelling down your body parts. This can happen either on both sides of the body or just on one side, depending on what structures are pushing on which nerves. Consider lower back pain, for example. Imagine that for the past few days you have experienced pain in your lower back after sitting for a few hours each day.

You figure the pain will go away so you don't change your daily routine in any way. After a few days the pain begins to travel down both sides of your buttocks, and eventually, when the pain hits your thigh, you become concerned. You remember reading that improper posture may produce uneven forces within a vertebral disc and that the disc can then push back on a nerve, causing pain. You also know that tight muscles add pressure to the nerves causing lower back pain and referring pain down your leg.

You begin to watch your posture and make positive changes: sitting up straight, using a lumbar roll, getting up from your chair once an hour, and performing the simple strengthening and stretching exercises covered in this book. The pain moves back up your body into your buttocks and in a few days has returned to your lower back. That is just what you want; when the pain centralizes, or returns to the source, it means that less pressure is being placed on the nerves and you are on the road to recovery. If you had noticed the pain continuing down your leg, you would have to be more aware of your posture. If the pain continued and you did not begin getting better within a few days, it would be wise to seek professional help (for example, seeing a physical therapist). Failure to improve might indicate that you need a hands-on approach to resolve your issue in addition to customized home exercises and postural positioning.

Remember, proper posture is not something that will come overnight, and it will take practice to improve upon. I hope you have gained new insight into the importance of proper body positioning and how it affects the body as a whole.

References

Baechle, Thomas R. and Roger W Earle: *Essentials of Strength Training and Conditioning.* National Strength and Conditioning Association, 3rd edition, 2008.

Levangie, Pamela and Cynthia Norkin: *Joint Structure and Function: A Comprehensive Analysis.* F.A Davis Co; 3rd edition, 2000.

McKenzie, Robin: *treat your own neck.* Spinal Publications New Zealand LTD; 4th edition, 2006.

Neumann, Donald A: *Kinesiology of the Musculoskeletal System. Foundations for Physical Rehabilitation.* Mosby, Inc., 2002.

Sahrmann, Shirley A: *Diagnosis and Treatment of Movement Impairment Syndromes:* Mosby Inc., 2001.

"Bad Posture—Number 2 of 4." Last modified Tuesday, July 29, 2008. http://posture-exercises.blogspot.com/2008/07/bad posture-number-2-of-4-lordotic.html

"How To Lift." Jonathan Cluett, M.D., About.com Guide. Last modified March 26, 2012. http://orthopedics.about.com/cs/backpain /ht/lift.htm

Horwitz, Dr. Steven. "Proper Shoe Fit." Last modified 1999. http://www.youcanbefit.com/shoes.html

"Importance of Sleep: Six reasons not to scrimp on sleep." Last modified 2012. http://www.health.harvard.edu/press_releases/importance_of_sleep_and_health

"Bad Posture—Number 4 of 4." Last modified Tuesday, July 29, 2008. http://posture-exercises.blogspot.com/2008/07/bad-posture-number-4-of-4-sway-back.html

"Improving Posture through Information and Direction." Last modified 2012.   http://posturereview.com/myPosture/kyphosisLordosisPosture.html

Wendy Bumgardner. "How to Walk—Walking Posture." Last modified July 29, 2011. http://walking.about.com/cs/beginners/a/howposture.htm